MAGIC

ARTS FOR HEALTH

Series Editor: Paul Crawford, Professor of Health Humanities, University of Nottingham, UK

The *Arts for Health* series offers a ground-breaking set of books that guide the general public, carers, and healthcare providers on how different arts can help people to stay healthy or improve their health and wellbeing.

Bringing together new information and resources underpinning the health humanities (that link health and social care disciplines with the arts and humanities), the books demonstrate the ways in which the arts offer people worldwide a kind of shadow health service – a non-clinical way to maintain or improve our health and wellbeing. The books are aimed at general readers along with interested arts' practitioners seeking to explore the health benefits of their work, health and social care providers and clinicians wishing to learn about the application of the arts for health, educators in arts, health and social care and organisations, carers and individuals engaged in public health or generating healthier environments. These easy-to-read, engaging short books help readers to understand the evidence about the value of arts for health and offer guidelines, case studies, and resources to make use of these non-clinical routes to a better life.

Other titles in the series:

Film	Steven Schlozman
Theatre	Sydney Cheek-O'Donnell
Singing	Yoon Irons and Grenville Hancox
Reading	Philip Davis
Drawing	Curie Scott
Photography	Susan Hogan
Storytelling	Michael Wilson
Music	Eugene Beresin

Forthcoming Titles

Painting	Javier Saaavedra, Samuel Arias, and Ana Rodríguez
Video	John Quin
Games	Sandra Danilovic
History	Anna Greenwood
Body Art	Brian Brown and Virginia Kuulei Berndt
Creative Writing	Mark Pearson and Helen Foster
Dancing	Noyale Colin and Kathryn Stamp

MAGIC

BY

RICHARD WISEMAN
University of Hertfordshire, UK

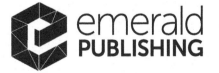

United Kingdom – North America – Japan – India
Malaysia – China

Emerald Publishing Limited
Howard House, Wagon Lane, Bingley BD16 1WA, UK

First edition 2023

Reprints and permissions service
Contact: www.copyright.com

British Library Cataloguing in Publication Data
A catalogue record for this book is available from the British Library

ISBN: 978-1-80455-613-9 (Print)
ISBN: 978-1-80455-610-8 (Online)
ISBN: 978-1-80455-612-2 (Epub)

INVESTOR IN PEOPLE

To Rex

CONTENTS

LIST OF FIGURES

ABOUT THE AUTHOR

Richard Wiseman holds Britain's only Professorship in the Public Understanding of Psychology at the University of Hertfordshire. He has published more than 100 academic papers, including those examining the psychology of magic, illusion, deception, luck, and self-development. He has also written popular psychology books that have sold over 3 million copies (including *The Luck Factor* and *59 Seconds*) and created illusion-based YouTube videos that have attracted more than 600 million views. He regularly gives keynote talks, is one of the most followed psychologists on Twitter, and the *Independent on Sunday* chose him as one of the top 100 people who make Britain a better place to live. Richard is a Member of the Inner Magic Circle, and acts as a creative consultant for high-profile stage and television projects. He was recently awarded the prestigious Golden Grolla Award for his work into psychology and illusion, and has been described by Elizabeth Loftus (Past President, Association for Psychological Science) as 'one of the world's most creative psychologists'.

FOREWORD: CREATIVE PUBLIC HEALTH

The 'Arts for Health' series aims to provide key information on how different arts and humanities practices can support, or even transform, health and wellbeing. Each book introduces a particular creative activity or resource and outlines its place and value in society, the evidence for its use in advancing health and wellbeing, and cases of how this works. In addition, each book provides useful links and suggestions to readers for following-up on these quick reads. We can think of this series as a kind of shadow health service – encouraging the use of the arts and humanities alongside all the other resources on offer to keep us fit and well.

Creative practices in the arts and humanities offer a fantastic, non-medical, but medically relevant way to improve the health and wellbeing of individuals, families, and communities. Intuitively, we know just how important creative activities are in maintaining or recovering our best possible lives. For example, imagine that we woke up tomorrow to find that all music, books, or films had to be destroyed, learn that singing, dancing, or theatre had been outlawed or that galleries, museums, and theatres had to close permanently; or, indeed, that every street had posters warning citizens of severe punishment for taking photographs, drawing, or writing. How would we feel? What would happen to our bodies and minds? How would we survive? Unfortunately, we have seen this kind of removal of creative activities from human society before and today many people remain terribly restricted in artistic expression and consumption.

I hope that this series adds a practical resource to the public. I hope people buy these little books as gifts for family and friends, or for hard-pressed healthcare professionals, to encourage them to revisit or to consider a creative path to living well. I hope that creative public health makes for a brighter future.

Professor Paul Crawford

ACKNOWLEDGEMENTS

I am grateful for the help and information supplied by the following people: Steven Bagienski, Jamie Balfour-Paul, Sadie Broome, Carlo Alfredo Clerici, David Copperfield, Gareth Foreman, Magic Gareth, Will Houstoun, Richard Kaufman, David Kaye, Helen Keen, Mike Lyons, Alan McCormack, Svetlana McMahon, Kevin McMahon, Lisa Mena, David Owen, Mary-Angela Papalaskari, Harrison Pravder, Brian South, Kevin Spencer, Scott Tokar, Michael Walton, and Darren Way. Also, special thanks to my wonderful interviewees: David Brookhouse, Julie Eng, David Gore, Marlies Greve, Richard McDougall, Mario Marchese, Rob van de Kamp, Tom Verner, and Marian Williamson. All of the interviews have been condensed and edited for clarity. And finally, to David Britland, Caroline Watt, and Jeff Wiseman for their invaluable help.

INTRODUCTION

When I was a child, my family and I used to visit my grandfather regularly. Although I enjoyed the requisite cup of tea and slice of fruitcake, the highlight of each trip involved him performing a wonderful illusion that he had learned during the Second World War. My grandfather began by handing me a marker pen and a Victorian penny, and then asking me to write my initials on the coin. He carefully placed the initialled coin onto his palm, closed his fingers around it, and then opened his hand to reveal that the coin had disappeared. Next, he reached under his chair and took out a metal tobacco tin that was about the size of a deck of cards. The tin was sealed tightly with several elastic bands, and he asked me to look inside. I carefully removed the bands, lifted the lid, and discovered that the tin contained an even smaller wooden box that was similarly sealed with more elastic bands. When I removed the second set of bands and opened the wooden box, I was amazed to discover my initialled coin.

For years, I pestered my grandfather to reveal the secret, and, like all good magicians, he steadfastly refused to spill the beans. Then, on my eighth birthday, he relented just a little, and told me that the solution was described in a book, and that that book was in my local library. At the time, I struggled with reading and so a library visit wasn't top of my agenda. Nevertheless, finding out the secret of the tobacco tin miracle was hugely appealing and so I went to the library and searched for books on magic. The books proved to be a portal into a wonderous world in which I was mesmerised by sensational stories of mysterious performers, fascinated by woodcuts illustrating complex sleight of hand, and spellbound by the secrets to hundreds of illusions. I was soon performing for my friends and family, and quickly discovered that magic often required a considerable amount of practice and hard work, and that watching a well-crafted illusion could be a transformative and fascinating experience.

I eventually uncovered the solution to the tobacco tin mystery. A few days later, I visited my grandfather and excitedly explained that I had completed my quest. He smiled, nodded, and then reached under his chair and handed me a secret object that played an essential role in the illusion. I have held onto that object for more than 40 years, and it currently resides in a display case in my office. Oh, and if you want to find out the secret to the mystery... then it's described in one of the magic books in your local library.

When I was about 12 years old, I joined my local magic club (The Mystic Ring in Luton) and continued my journey into the art of conjuring. I found out that there is more to magic than meets the eye. Unlike many performing arts, magic doesn't require spectators to suspend their disbelief, and seeing the impossible apparently made possible can induce a unique sense of awe, astonishment, and wonder (Lamont, 2017; Leddington, 2016). Magicians and academics have argued that this amazing experience helps to explain the universal appeal of magic and has the power to awaken people's dreams and to expand their horizons (Wiseman & Watt, 2022).

In my early teens, I started to perform at children's parties and made notes about each of my shows in a little blue book. I have that book in front of me right now, and so I know that my first performance was on 3 April 1979, that I was paid three pounds, and that one child noticed that I had an egg hidden under my arm at the start of the show. During my twenties, I became a member of The Magic Circle, performed street magic in London's Covent Garden, and travelled to America to work at The Magic Castle, a prestigious private magic club in Hollywood.

Over time, I became interested in the fascinating relationship between magic and psychology. Good magicians understand how to control audiences' attention, how to encourage them to make certain assumptions, and how to play with their memory. Academics have long been interested in these topics, with some of the earliest work dating back to the turn of the twentieth century.

For instance, in 1894, the French psychologist Alfred Binet investigated whether the hand really is quicker than the eye by having magicians perform sleight of hand in front of a camera that took several photographs of their movements in rapid succession (Binet, 1894). Similarly, in 1896, Joseph Jastrow conducted experiments into the dexterity and mental skills with two famous illusionists of his day, Alexander Herrmann and Harry Kellar (Jastrow, 1896). Inspired by this type of work, I eventually enrolled for an undergraduate degree in psychology at University College London (chosen, in part, because it is close to The Magic Circle) and then completed a doctorate in the psychology of deception at the University of Edinburgh. Shortly afterwards, I joined the University of Hertfordshire, where I am now a professor of psychology.

Much of my early research examined why magic works and involved studying the psychology employed by experienced magicians (Lamont & Wiseman, 1999), exploring whether psychology can inspire new illusions (Lamont & Wiseman, 2003; Wiseman & Lamont, 2003), and examining how conjurors and fake psychics fool their audiences (Wiseman et al., 2003; Wiseman & Morris, 1995). In the last decade, this area has attracted the attention of many more academics (for a review, see Kuhn, 2019). Then, in 2008, I started to expand the focus of this work and to examine the therapeutic and educational benefits of watching and learning magic (Derbyshire, 2008; Paton, 2008).

I soon discovered that magic is used to help people in a surprisingly wide variety of settings. For instance, hospital magicians aid patients' recovery, occupational therapists employ magic to boost motor skills and coordination, counsellors conjure up key life skills, and teachers perform illusions to promote attention and curiosity. These activities are highly practical and often easier to implement than interventions associated with other performing arts. Whereas plays, dance, and concerts often need to be staged in relatively formal settings, people can be shown or perform magic almost anywhere. Whilst learning to play a musical instrument or memorising a script can be difficult and time consuming, some illusions can be mastered very quickly. Plays, dance routines, and music concerts often involve lengthy and fixed forms of performance, whereas magic is highly flexible, can be adapted to suit individuals' needs and abilities, and is easily tailored to any length of show. Also, from an economic perspective, purchasing a musical instrument can be costly, whilst lots of illusions just involve inexpensive everyday objects.

More recently, several academics (myself included) reviewed research examining the efficacy of magic-based interventions and discovered that most of the work has yielded positive findings (Bagienski & Kuhn, 2019, 2020; Lam et al., 2017; Wiseman & Watt, 2018, 2020). In addition, I conducted several studies in the area, examining, for instance, how magic boosts creativity, enhances student engagement, and encourages critical thinking (Wiseman et al., 2020, 2021). I also teamed up with experienced performers to create illusions and shows that encourage children to tackle challenging tasks, to persevere when the going gets tough, and to learn how to deal with negative emotions (Wiseman & Kaye, 2020). Together, this work convinced me that magic has an important, and possibly unique, role to play in enhancing wellbeing, health, and education.

This book presents a comprehensive examination of the relationship between magic and wellbeing, and addresses two main issues.

Firstly, magic has been employed in a disparate range of therapeutic and educational contexts, and these performers and practitioners are often unaware of each other's work. This book brings together this diverse activity and unifies it into a single discipline of Applied Magic.

Secondly, magic tends to be neglected in discussions about the performing arts and health. This may be due to the secretive nature of conjuring, the mistaken belief that magic isn't an art form, or that work in the area is often published in relatively obscure books and journals. Whatever the explanation, many people are unaware of the benefits of watching and learning magic. This book aims to address this issue and to bring the power of Applied Magic to the attention of a wide range of practitioners, performers, and academics.

Chapter One takes a brief look at the subculture of magic and describes some of the illusions that are often used in therapeutic and educational work. Each of the following chapters then explores one of the three main types of Applied Magic. Chapter Two examines how magic is employed within a medical setting, Chapter Three investigates how it's used to build life skills, and Chapter Four reviews work into magic and education. Each of these chapters begins by describing some of the most successful programmes in the area and highlighting especially interesting ideas. Hopefully, practitioners and performers will find this material informative and inspirational. The chapters then review research that has assessed the efficacy of this work. These studies are important as they ensure that the area is evidence-based and help to attract participants, institutions, collaborators, and funders. At the end of each chapter, there are in-depth interviews with experienced practitioners involved in this area, exploring how they became involved in the field, how they go about their work, and how they overcome challenges and issues. Finally, the Conclusion outlines seven ways in which Applied Magic can grow and develop in the future.

I hope that you find our time together enjoyable, informative, and magical.

1

A PEEK BEHIND THE CURTAIN

This chapter presents a brief guide to the subculture of magic, takes an in-depth look at the types of illusions employed in therapeutic and educational work, and concludes with some general advice for those starting out in conjuring.

THE SUBCULTURE OF MAGIC

Conjurors are a naturally secretive bunch and so the public tend to have little insight into the world of magic. Here's a brief guide to this intriguing subculture.

First, magic has a long lasting and universal appeal. Records from ancient cultures contain accounts of magic shows, with some of the earliest descriptions appearing in works by the legendary Greek philosopher Plato and the great Roman scholar Seneca. Throughout history, magicians have continued to astound people, and even the dramatic rise of science and technology has done nothing to dent the enduring popularity of this unusual performing art. Nowadays, famous magicians still attract huge audiences to their lives shows and videos of illusions attract millions of views on social media.

Second, magic is a small, well organised, and close-knit community. Many large towns and cities have a local magic club where members will meet, perform for each other, and offer encouragement and criticism (usually the latter). In addition, many countries have a national magic society, such as The Magic Circle in Britain and The Society of American Magicians in the USA. At a global level, The International Brotherhood of Magicians currently boasts thousands of members in more than 80 countries. Lots of these clubs and societies regularly stage shows for the public, as well as organising conferences and conventions for magicians. Some of these events are surprisingly large with, for example, the Blackpool Magic Convention attracting more than 4,000 magicians each year. There are also individuals and businesses that sell magic, with many magic shops offering lessons to beginners and providing a meeting place for magicians.

Third, magicians have produced a vast amount of literature about their art. Reginald Scot's *The Discoverie of Witchcraft* was published in 1584 and is widely seen as the first English language book to contain detailed descriptions of magic tricks. Since then, magicians have written thousands of books for their fellow deceivers, including those containing instructions for performing sleight of hand, plans of magical apparatus and discussions about the theory of magic. In addition, they have published long-running magazines that are replete with new illusions, reports of conventions, advertisements, and profiles of well-known performers. Organisations like The Magic Circle and The Magic Castle maintain immense and impressive libraries, and most recently. The Conjuring Arts Research Center in New York created an online database of key publications that currently contains over 2.5 million pages of material.

Appendix 1 contains information about recommended books, magazines, organisations, and shops.

SOME TRICKS OF THE TRADE

Performing magic can be challenging because it often involves the careful handling of apparatus, learning difficult sleight of hand, remembering the order of a complex series of actions, and creating entertaining presentations. Because of this, it can take years of practise, hard work, and dedication to master. In contrast, most of the illusions used in Applied Magic must be suitable for beginners and so they tend to involve everyday objects, are relatively easy to learn, can be performed in many settings, and are easily adapted to meet individual needs and abilities. This section describes several illusions that are frequently employed in this work. These have been chosen to highlight the diversity of material available to performers and practitioners, and to illustrate a range of therapeutic and educational benefits. Each description contains four subsections: Effect, Method, Presentation and Notes.

Effect: This part contains a relatively brief description of an impossible happening. Some magicians have argued that effects can be classified into several categories, such as appearances (e.g. a rabbit being produced from a top hat), vanishes (illusionist David Copperfield making the Statue of Liberty disappear), transpositions (my grandfather making a coin magically move from his hand to a sealed tin), transformations (a playing card changing into a coin or a person transforming into an animal), penetrations (solid metal rings linking together or a person penetrating through a solid sheet of glass), levitations and suspensions (a ball floating into the air or a person flying across the stage), restorations (two pieces of rope becoming one or a person being sawn in half and then restored), and extraordinary mental feats (a performer reading someone's mind, influencing their behaviour or predicting the future).

Method: The method explains the secret behind the illusion, including the apparatus required, any secret preparation, and the actions carried out during the performance.

Presentation: Magicians have developed many ways of presenting their illusions, with some performers taking themselves very seriously, others adopting a far more comedic approach, and a few even pretending that they can work genuine miracles. This section describes possible plots, storylines, and scripting.

Notes: This section contains additional information about the illusion, including variations of the effect and method, the way in which it can be used in a therapeutic and educational context, and credits to those who helped to create or to inspire it.

Is That Your Card?

Effect: A spectator selects a playing card from the deck, looks at it and replaces their card back into the deck. The deck is cut several times. The magician then deals out each card from the top of the deck one at a time and apparently uses their intuition to correctly identify the chosen card.

Method:

Apparatus: A deck of playing cards (and the illusion will even work if some of the cards are missing).

Preparation: Before starting, secretly look at the playing card on the bottom of the deck and remember it. This is known as a key card.

Performance: Spread out the playing cards face down between your hands, and ask the spectator to take a card and remember it. Next, close the spread of cards and ask the spectator to place their card on top of the deck. Cut the deck by splitting it roughly in half and placing the top part underneath the bottom part. This ensures that the key card is now on top of the chosen card. Hand the deck to the spectator and ask them to carry out the same actions, cutting the deck as many times as they like. Their chosen card will apparently be lost in the deck, but it will still be directly below the key card.

Next, deal the top card of the deck face up onto the table. Then repeat this same move with the second card, then the third card, and so on as you make your way through the deck. At some point, you will see the key card. When this happens, stop, and say that you have a strange feeling about the next card. Deal the next card face up, and it will be the spectator's chosen card. If the key card happens to be the final card that you turn over, the spectator's chosen card was the first card that you dealt.

This illusion requires practise as it's important that you don't forget the key card, and are able to smoothly spread out the cards, reform the deck, and cut it. The more that you carry out these movements, the more comfortable you will be when performing the illusion.

Presentation: Saying that you have an intuitive feeling about the next card is only one of many possible presentations. To make the illusion more interactive and fun, you could say that you can detect the spectator's fingerprints on the back of their card, and then examine the back of each card before you turn it over. Or you could explain that most people unconsciously wiggle their nose when they see their card and then study the spectator's face after each card is revealed (pretending to detect a slight nose wiggle when you deal out their card). This trick can be shown to just one person or a small group, and it can be performed with alphabet cards, top trumps, happy family cards, etc..

Notes: Within a therapeutic and educational context, this illusion is often taught to people to help to boost their cognitive skills (recalling the key card and remembering the correct sequence of events), to improve their hand movements and co-ordination (handling the cards), and to enhance their social skills (interacting with the spectator and developing an entertaining presentation).

The Jumping Band

Effect: The magician places a rubber band around their first and second fingers and then closes their hand into a fist. When the magician opens their fist, the band magically jumps to their third and fourth fingers.

Method:
Apparatus: A rubber band that is about the size of a bracelet.
Preparation: Prior to the performance, you will need to place the rubber band on your fingers in a certain way. Begin by putting the band around the first and second fingers of one hand (Fig. 1), and then, with your other hand, pull the band towards yourself (Fig. 2).

Next, fold all four fingers inside the band (Fig. 3), and then release the band so that it lies across your fingernails (Fig. 4). Now you are ready to perform the trick.
Performance: Show the back of your hand to the spectator. It will look like the rubber band is just around the base of your first and second fingers. Next, say: One, Two, Three ... Go. As you say the word Go, quickly open your hand, pushing the band up with all four fingernails (Fig. 5). The band will magically appear to jump to the base of your other two fingers.

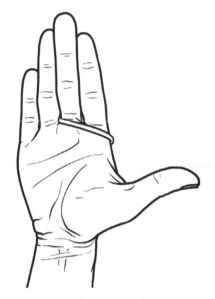

Fig. 1.   Put the Band Around the First and Second Fingers of One Hand.

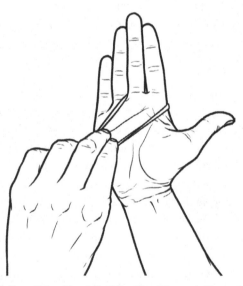

Fig. 2.   With Your Other Hand, Pull The Band Towards Yourself.

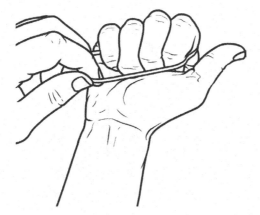

Fig. 3.   Fold All Four Fingers Inside the Band.

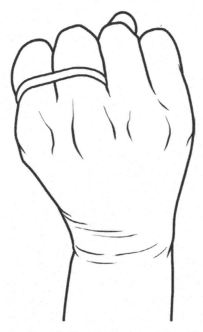

Fig. 4.   Release the Band So That It Lies Across Your Fingernails.

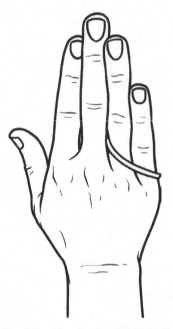

Fig. 5.   Open Your Hand, Pushing the Band Up With Your Fingernails.

This illusion requires practise, but it's easy to keep the rubber band in your pocket and to spend a few moments each day rehearsing the movements.

Presentation: The Jumping Band is especially well-suited to storytelling. You could, for instance, say that the band wants to compete in the forthcoming rubber band Olympics. Suggest that it's training for the long jump but first needs to warm up with some stretches (stretch the band a few times). Next, place the band over your first two fingers and carry out the secret move as you close your hand. Then say that the band is ready for the big jump and countdown by saying 'On your marks, Get set, Go.' When you say the word 'Go', open your hand and the band will jump across to your other two fingers. To add some drama, you could have the band fail to jump the first few times (by placing the band around your first and second fingers but not carrying out the secret move when you close your hand) before being successful.

Notes: The Jumping Band was invented by British conjuror Stanley Collins and published in a magazine called *The Magician Monthly* more than a hundred years ago. Since then, magicians have developed many variations of the illusion. For example, rather than just opening their hand, some magicians quickly open and then close their hand, masking these actions by moving their hand up and down at the same time. A magician named Okito twisted a second rubber band around the tops of all four fingers and discovered that the trick still works. Another variation involves placing a second, different coloured, band around the third and fourth fingers, and using the same type of move to make the two bands change places.

The illusion encourages a series of skills, including empathy (making the illusion interesting and entertaining), persistence and practise (rehearsing the secret move), problem solving (figuring out why it works), and creativity (exploring variations). The Jumping Band can also help to convey key life lessons by, for example, developing a storyline that highlights the importance of perseverance and resilience.

The Magic Pencil

Effect: The magician makes a pencil magically stick to their hand.

Method:
Apparatus: This trick only requires a pencil. There is no secret preparation.
Performance: Place the pencil in your left fist, which should be held vertically with your thumb on top. Ensure that the ends stick out above and below the fist. Make sure that the fingers of your left hand are facing the spectator and that they can see that you are only holding the pencil. Next, move your hand around in front of you, such that the back of the hand is now facing the spectator. Place your right hand around your left wrist, and secretly extend your right first finger so that it goes inside your left fist and pushes the pencil against the palm. Finally, open the fingers of your left hand as far as possible and it will appear as if the pencil is magically stuck to the palm of your hand. You can even shake your hand to show that the pencil is firmly attached. Finally, reverse the movements and remove the pencil.

Presentation: This illusion is not hugely fooling but it's simple to perform, and is often presented in an informal way to create a sense of fun. In terms of a possible presentation, you might explain that you kept losing your pencil and so have created a way of making it magically stick to your hand.

Notes: This illusion can be performed with many objects, such as a pen, a straw, or a wand. Health practitioners sometimes use it to familiarise younger patients with medical equipment (such as a spatula or tongue depressor), and dentists can perform it with a toothbrush to gain children's attention before talking about the importance of oral hygiene.

Mind To Mind

Effect: This illusion is performed for a group of spectators. The magician first assembles five random objects and then leaves the room for a few minutes, having told the group to choose one of them. Upon returning, the magician asks one spectator to think about the chosen object. They then apparently read the spectator's mind and correctly identify the object.

Method:
Apparatus: This illusion can be performed with any five objects.
Preparation: Unlike most magic, this illusion uses a stooge. Before the performance begins, secretly take one person in the group aside and ask them if they are willing to help. Explain that during the illusion, you will place five objects in a line on a table. Ask your stooge to mentally number the objects, starting with the object on their left, from one to five. You will then leave the room, having asked the group to choose one of the objects in your absence. Upon your return, the stooge should use their right hand to secretly signal the chosen object by showing the corresponding number of fingers. If, for instance, object number one is chosen, the stooge should hold out one finger. However, if object number five is chosen, they should show four fingers and their thumb. Ask the stooge to make the signal as subtle as possible by casually keeping their hand on their chair or down by their side.

Performance: Ask the group to place any five objects on a table and arrange them into a line. Explain that you will leave the room for a few minutes and that during this time, the group needs to choose one of the objects. When you return, ask one person in the group (not your stooge) to concentrate on the chosen object. Glance at the secret signal from your stooge and then dramatically reveal the chosen object.

Presentation: This illusion can be presented in many ways. For example, you might say that you are able to detect the chosen object based on tiny unconscious movements made by members of the group as you name each object. This involves lots of people and so feels more inclusive. Or you can ask someone to imagine the chosen object, pretend to enter their mind and say that you are seeing a strange image (e.g. 'I am seeing a garden gnome riding on the back of a flamingo...'), and end by linking this image to the chosen object ('... hold on, the flamingo has something around its neck...it's the key').

Notes: Because this illusion involves two people working together, it can be used to build trust and to illustrate the value of collaborating. The illusion also presents an opportunity for older participants to team up with younger friends and family, and thus promotes intergenerational connectivity.

The idea of a stooge secretly signalling information to the magician has been around for a very long time and is even described in Reginald Scot's 1584 book, *The Discoverie Of Witchcraft*.

The Twenty-One Card Trick

Effect: A spectator chooses a playing card from a packet of 21 cards. The magician then deals the cards face up into three columns, and the spectator indicates which column contains their chosen card. The magician collects the cards and deals them out again. This procedure is repeated a few times, and the magician eventually reveals the chosen card.

Method:
Apparatus: This illusion is performed with 21 playing cards. There is no secret preparation.

Performance: Ask the spectator to look through the cards and to choose one. Hold the packet of cards face down and deal out the top three cards face up in a row, moving left to right. Deal out the next row in the same way, and continue doing this until you have three columns, each of which contains seven face up cards.

Next, ask the spectator to indicate which of the three columns contains their chosen card. Push each column into a pile, being careful not to mix up their order, and then pick up the three piles, ensuring that the chosen pile goes between the other two. This should be carried out quickly to ensure that your spectator doesn't notice that you are stacking the columns in a particular order.

Turn the entire packet face down and again deal out three columns of seven cards, left to right. Ask your spectator to indicate which column now contains their card, carefully make the three columns into three piles, and pick up the piles ensuring that the chosen column again goes between the other two. Repeat this fascinating process one last time. Now for the grand finale. Turn the deck face down and spell out the letters in the phrase 'Your card is', dealing the top card face up as you spell each letter. The next card that you deal out will be the spectator's card.

Presentation: An alternative presentation of the trick involves the spectator appearing to perform the magic. After the cards have been collected up the final time, hand the deck to the spectator and ask them to deal off cards as they spell out the magic word. When presented within an educational context, students can be asked to try to discover the mathematical principle underpinning the trick. The illusion can also be used to convey a range of educational and health messages by replacing the magic phrase with something like 'Brush teeth' or 'Never bully.'

Notes: This illusion has a long history, with one of the earliest versions appearing in a 1593 manuscript written by Italian magician Horatio Galasso. Galasso notes that the effect works with any odd number of cards and presents a version with 15 cards, with the chosen card appearing at the 8th position.

The Amazing Straw

Effect: The magician balances a plastic drinking straw horizontally on the top of a bottle and then uses telekinetic powers to make the straw magically spin around.

Method:
Apparatus: You will need a plastic or glass bottle, and a plastic drinking straw. The illusion works best with a bottle that has a cap on it.
Preparation: Before you begin, place the bottle on the table, secretly rub the plastic straw on some wool clothing or a piece of cloth, and then balance it horizontally on the top of the bottle.
Performance: Place your hands a few inches away from either end of the straw and move them around. Nothing will happen because your hands are too far away from the straw. Now announce that you will use your magical powers to make the straw rotate. Place your hands close to the ends of the straw, being careful not to touch it, and again move them in a circular direction. Static electricity will ensure that the straw rotates around on the top of the bottle.

Presentation: Rather than demonstrating your psychic powers, the same effect can be used to discover whether a spectator has paranormal powers. To achieve this, ask a spectator to carefully move their hands around the straw and it will move.

Notes: Teachers and lecturers can perform this illusion in science lessons to promote curiosity and engagement. After the demonstration, students can be challenged to figure out the secret behind the trick and to test their ideas by performing the demonstration under different conditions.

The Book of Spells

Effect: The magician flicks through a notebook and shows that all the pages are blank. They then utter the magic words 'Bring Me Magic' and suddenly the notebook becomes full of strange drawings and mystical spells.

Method:

Apparatus: Making the special notebook will take some time. First, obtain a notebook that is soft backed, has identical front and back covers, and contains pages that are made from quite thick paper through which the ink can't be seen. Second, use a pencil to lightly number the pages as if the notebook were a regular novel. Third, turn over page 1 and place a pencil dot on page 3, then turn over 2 pages and place a dot on page 7, then continue the sequence of turning over 2 pages and placing a dot throughout the book. The dotted pages should be numbered 3, 7, 11, 15, etc. Fourth, carefully trim about 4mm off the long edge of every page that has a dot on it. This will result in each page having one of two widths, alternating wide, narrow, wide, narrow, throughout the notebook. Finally, add text and drawings on pages 2 and 3, skip pages 4 and 5, add more drawings and text to pages 6 and 7, so on throughout the notebook. As you are producing a book of spells, it's good to make the drawings and text look mysterious and strange.

Performance: Rest the spine of the notebook on your left hand and use your right hand to flick through the pages. Because of the arrangement of wide and narrow pages, the notebook will appear to be completely blank. Next, say the magic words 'Bring Me Magic'. Turn the notebook over end to end as you say each of these three words. This will reverse the notebook, such that the back cover is now facing you. However, as the front and back covers are identical, your spectators will not notice the difference. Flick through the book again and this time the pages will appear to be full of mysterious spells.

Presentation: This illusion can be presented in many ways. For instance, you might want to begin by saying that you first need to brush up on your magical skills and explain that you have a book of spells. You show that the pages of the notebook are empty, make the spells appear and then apparently use one of the spells in your next illusion. In addition to saying the magic word, you can also make the presentation more interactive by having the spectator blow on the book to make the spells appear (for this reason, this type of book is often referred to as a blow book). Health practitioners can use the book to make the instructions for a procedure magically appear, and child counsellors can use it to help impart important life lessons by, for example, writing negative emotions on the pages and then making them vanish.

Notes: This illusion illustrates how magic tricks encourage maker skills. Magicians have created more complex versions of the book using different sets of images, such that the pages might begin blank, and then black and white drawings appear, and then these images transform into full colour drawings. This is another illusion that has a long history, with Reginald Scot describing a version in 1584.

Through a Postcard

Effect: This is more of a puzzle than an illusion. The magician announces that they will place their head through a postcard and then performs this seemingly impossible feat.

Method:
Apparatus: You will need a postcard and a pair of scissors.
Performance: The method involves a clever topological principle. First, fold the postcard in half and cut along the vertical lines shown in Fig. 6. Make sure that you cut both sides of the fold.

Second, carefully unfold the postcard and cut along the dotted line (Fig. 7). Make sure that you don't cut through the two end strips.

Finally, gently pull on the ends of the postcard, and you will find that it opens out to form a large chain of connected strips, which can then easily be placed over your head (Fig. 8).

Presentation: This item can be used to teach topology, to show how apparently complex problems often have surprisingly simple solutions, and to demonstrate how it's sometimes possible to achieve the seemingly impossible.

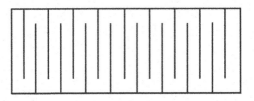

Fig. 6. Fold and Cut the Postcard.

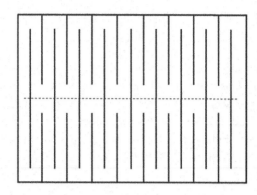

Fig. 7. Open and the Postcard and Make the Final Cut Along the Dotted Line.

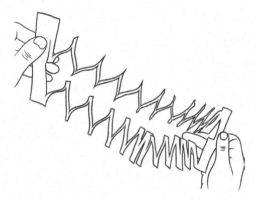

Fig. 8. Gently Pull on the Ends and Open the Postcard.

SHOPPING FOR MAGIC

The following list presents brief descriptions of several illusions that are widely available in magic shops and especially well-suited to Applied Magic.

D'lite: Invented by Roger Mayfarth, this highly visual illusion involves the magician apparently plucking a bright light out of thin air, throwing the light from hand to hand, placing it in their ear and mouth, and much more.

Zig-zag rope: The magician threads a thick piece of rope through two plastic blocks, appears to cut it in half by sliding the blocks apart, and then magically restores the rope. The original version of this illusion was called Clean Cut and invented by Hiroshi Kondo.

Colour vision: The spectator is given a cube with six coloured sides and is then asked to choose a colour and to place the cube inside an opaque box. Nevertheless, the magician is instantly able to divine the chosen colour. This illusion was invented by Martin Sunshine.

Professor's nightmare: In this now classic illusion, three ropes of different lengths magically become the same length and then transform back into three different lengths. This trick is widely credited to Bob Carver.

Mental epic: Sometimes called the Mental Prediction Board, this trick was invented by Hen Fetsch. The magician shows a board containing six spaces, writes predictions in three of them, and covers the predictions up. The spectator makes a series of choices, and these are written in the remaining spaces. When the magician's predictions are revealed, they all match the spectator's choices.

Sponge balls: Almost all magic shops sell sets of sponge balls, and magicians have created lots of illusions in which these balls appear, vanish, and jump from hand to hand. These routines are a good introduction to relatively simple sleight of hand and are fun to perform. Although magician Albert Goshman popularised sponge ball magic, the original idea was first described by Jesse J. Lybarger in the 1920s.

Svengali Deck: This deck of cards is cleverly gimmicked and allows beginners to perform a series of amazing effects. Some magic historians have argued that the deck was invented more than 100 years ago by American magician Burling Hull.

GENERAL ADVICE

Try not to repeat an illusion: Spectators might ask you to repeat a trick or to show it to their friends. This is often a compliment because it suggests that they were bamboozled and want a second chance to figure out the illusion or would like their friends to have the same magical experience. Although you might be tempted to perform the illusion again, this is usually a bad idea because spectators will have a much better chance of working out the secret. There are exceptions to this rule because there are some illusions that are specially designed to be repeated, but they usually involve changing the method each time. In general, if a spectator asks to see an illusion again, offer to show them something even more amazing.

Resist the urge to reveal methods: People will often ask you to explain the secret to an illusion, in part because they assume that it will be fascinating and complex. In fact, such secrets are often surprisingly simple. For example, in the illusions described above, the magician identified a chosen playing card by just remembering the bottom card of the deck and appeared to read people's minds with the help of a stooge. Discovering the secret to an illusion often results in a sense of disappointment and, more importantly, means that it will no longer elicit a sense of wonder or joy. Because of this, magicians tend to avoid telling people how their illusions work. Joining magic societies usually involves taking an oath of secrecy, and exposure is generally frowned upon, although there are exceptions, such as when a trick is being used by a fake psychic or con artist. When asked to explain the secret to an illusion, try deflecting the question with a light-hearted comment (e.g. 'I have no idea, I think it's magic'.) Although taking an oath of secrecy isn't practical for this book, please respect the magician's code and refrain from telling people the secrets described in this chapter.

Practise, practise, practise: Even the simplest illusions require practise and rehearsal. Sometimes you might be tempted to perform an illusion for people immediately after finding out the secret. Try to avoid this temptation and instead find the time to practise the required movements and to devise an entertaining presentation. When rehearsing an illusion, it's often helpful to practise in front of a mirror so that you can see how everything looks from the spectator's point of view. Once you have mastered the moves and words, try showing it to a few close friends and family. If this goes well, you are ready to perform for others.

Less is more: When people start to immerse themselves in the world of magic, they often want to learn as many illusions as possible. Instead, try to focus on learning how to perform a small number of tricks properly. David Devant was one of the most famous magicians in Britain around the turn of the last century, and once described meeting a young conjuror who proudly declared that he knew about 300 tricks. Devant explained that he only knew eight tricks but had learned to how to perform them extremely well.

Dealing with nerves: Even the most experienced magicians can become nervous when they perform. Practising and rehearsal helps to lower nerves, as does the actor's trick of telling yourself that you are excited rather than nervous. However, the most effective way of building confidence is to perform as much as possible.

Be prepared: Magic can go wrong, and so it's important to try to avoid common pitfalls and to think about what you will do if something fails. For example, a spectator might derail a card trick by forgetting their chosen card. If you are performing for a group of people, you can prevent this by asking the spectator to show their chosen card to other people. Alternatively, you might have a rubber band break or forget the identity of a key card during a card trick. Again, these issues can be prevented by having several replacement bands in your pocket and always using the same key card.

SUMMARY

This chapter briefly explored the secretive subculture of magic, including its history, literature, and organisation. It then presented an in-depth look at several illusions that are often used in Applied Magic, including how to put your head through a postcard, how to make a pencil stick to your hand, and how to fill a blank notebook with mysterious symbols. These illusions were carefully chosen because they are relatively simple to learn and illustrate a range of therapeutic and educational benefits. Finally, the chapter outlined some general guidance for trainee magicians. To start your journey into the wonderful world of magic, try performing some of these illusions for your friends and family.

2

MEDICAL MAGIC

One key area of Applied Magic involves using illusions to help patients within a medical context. This chapter explores the background of this area, describes key initiatives, reviews research that has assessed this work, and presents interviews with experienced practitioners.

BACKGROUND

Born in 1895 in a small Welsh village, Richard Pitchford became fascinated with conjuring at an early age. When the First World War broke out, he signed up, was sent to France, and spent spare time in the trenches practising sleight of hand with playing cards. During the Battle of the Somme, a shell detonated close to Pitchford and caused him to lose consciousness. As he was suffering from severe shell shock, he was eventually moved to a British hospital and spent a large amount of time manipulating playing cards to help aid his recovery. After being discharged in 1919, Pitchford developed a highly successful magic act in which he played the role of a tipsy aristocrat who was bewildered by playing cards and other objects inexplicably appearing at his fingertips. Adopting the stage name Cardini, Pitchford amazed audiences across the globe, and is now widely considered to have been one of the world's most highly skilled magicians. Pitchford frequently described how practicing magic in the hospital aided his recovery, and how he considered it to be an early form of occupational therapy.

Magician and illustrator Charles Folkard also recognised how conjuring could promote the wellbeing of soldiers during the First World War. In 1915, he adopted the pseudonym Draklof (Folkard spelt backwards) and wrote two booklets (both entitled *Tricks for the Trenches and Wards*) describing illusions that can be performed with everyday objects (Draklof, 1915a, 1915b).

During the Second World War, magician and psychiatrist Douglas Kelley pioneered the use of magic as therapy at the New York State Psychiatric Institute. In a lengthy article, Kelley (1940) outlined the benefits of this approach, noting how learning magic promoted patients' sense of mastery and how exploring different ways of presenting illusions encouraged the imagination. He also described how magic aids social interaction, noting that when people discover that someone is a magician, they frequently ask to see a trick.

In the 1950s, magician Charles Reiss was hospitalised for war-related injuries and started to perform magic for staff and visitors (Lopez, 1957). Certain that his fellow patients would benefit from learning magic, Reiss taught them a few illusions. Inspired by the positive results, Reiss initiated similar projects in other hospitals and eventually persuaded The Society of American Magicians to form the National Committee for Therapy Through Magic. As far as I am aware, this committee no longer exists.

Since then, health practitioners and performers have created several magic-based initiatives. This work involves magician–practitioner collaborations, magicians working alone, and health professionals learning to perform magic.

MAGICIAN–PRACTITIONER COLLABORATIONS

Project Magic

In 1981, legendary American illusionist David Copperfield created Project Magic. This pioneering programme involves magicians and health professionals working together to create interventions that promote patient wellbeing. The programme was developed with the help of occupational therapist Julie DeJean and was endorsed by The American Occupational Therapy Association. The Project Magic website describes how the programme was adopted by hospitals in nearly every state across America and spread to many other countries.

In the Project Magic handbook, highly skilled magicians David Copperfield and Richard Kaufman (2002) describe 50 illusions that are well suited to this work, ranging from magic with everyday objects to large stage items that can be constructed from cardboard boxes. The handbook also explains how to maximise the therapeutic value of each illusion and classifies illusions according to whether they help to improve motor, cognitive, or social skills. For example, it describes how The Jumping Band (see Chapter One) improves both fine and gross motor control and notes how it can be practised with increasingly thick elastic bands to help to increase finger strength and flexibility. The handbook also offers a wealth of practical advice, including how practitioners and magicians can contact one another and how to choose illusions that best match patients' needs and abilities.

My Magic Hands

Founded in 2004, this Canadian programme was created by Julie Eng and David Ben from the Magicana organisation. The programme teaches magic to groups of children and young adults, usually lasts between six and eight weeks, and is delivered by a professional magician supported by occupational therapists or volunteers from a partner organisation. This structure provides participants with individual instruction and a positive role model. During the sessions, the participants are provided with the apparatus required to perform various illusions and introduced to other relevant performance skills, including scripting, stagecraft, and choreography. At the end of the programme, the participants perform a show for their friends and family. My Magic Hands has been delivered in a variety of medical contexts, including at a rehabilitation hospital to support children recovering from brain injuries and at a summer camp for children with cancer.

Breathe Magic Intensive Therapy Programme

This British initiative was created in 2010 by barrister and magician David Owen and social entrepreneur Yvonne Farquharson, with magician Richard McDougall joining them in designing the programme. It aims to help young people with hemiplegia (a weakness or paralysis affecting one side of the body) by teaching them magic to boost their motor skills, cognitive abilities, and self-confidence. This support is tailored to each child's abilities and needs, with much of the work aiming to make repetitive therapeutic movements more meaningful by incorporating them into carefully designed illusions. These sessions are often delivered during a 10-day magic therapy course and follow-up workshops that are led by highly skilled magicians, including Richard McDougall, Will Houstoun, Laura London, Jon M. Armstrong, Harry De Cruz, James Freedman, Edward Hilsum, Christopher Howell, and Jez Rose. During these group sessions, a magician acts as a teacher and occupational therapists provide one-to-one support for participants. For an in-depth look at this work, see my interview with Richard McDougall later in this chapter.

More recently, Breathe has also begun to explore how magic might help to improve mental health. These six-to-eight-week programmes are based around participant's needs and abilities and use magic to enhance cognitive functioning and memory, to boost confidence and self-belief, and to improve social skills. This work has involved several groups of participants, including children at a mental health inpatient unit at London's Great Ormond Street Hospital and women experiencing antenatal and postnatal mental health issues. As is always the case in Breathe's work, the illusions were developed in collaboration between health professionals and magicians, including Breathe magicians Will Houstoun and Richard McDougall. Houstoun believes that one key benefit of this approach involves increased empowerment. Hospital patients often find themselves in a relatively powerless situation where they are encouraged to undergo prescribed treatments and to follow the advice of medical staff. Performing magic provides them with a safe and playful context within which they can exert authority and control.

In 2020, I teamed up with The Good Thinking Society to create an award that celebrated positive uses of magic. Our first Good Magic award went to Breathe to support their valuable work.

MAGICIANS WORKING ALONE

Open Heart Magic

In 2003, American magician Michael Walton set up Open Heart Magic (Hart & Walton, 2010). This initiative involves magicians working independently on children's wards in hospitals, with volunteer performers being required to complete an extensive 12-week training programme that focuses on several key issues, including ensuring patient safety, choosing magic that is appropriate to patients' abilities and needs, and understanding hospital regulations. It also emphasises using magic in a manner that is interactive and maximises the positive effect on children dealing with the stress of serious disease and treatment. Before being allowed to work on a ward, each volunteer must learn specific magic tricks and understand how to perform these in a range of contexts, including working in isolation rooms and with children who have been traumatised by their situation. This is completed through Magic University, which includes performance tests, immersion roleplay evaluations, and written exams. Open Heart Magic currently operates on paediatric and patient wards within 12 hospitals around America, including the Cleveland Clinic and Ann & Robert H. Lurie Children's Hospital of Chicago. The organisation encourages the magicians to work with patients, their siblings, and parents. This inclusive approach ensures that patients benefit from experiencing magic and seeing their parents having a good time, and that their siblings receive some much-needed attention.

Magic Care

Founded in the Netherlands in 2005 by four experts in different aspects of magic therapy (Rob van de Kamp, Igor de Kort, Marlies Greve, and Wim van Dokkum), Magic Care magicians perform and teach magic to children in hospitals. Health practitioners first identify children who will benefit from the initiative, and then two magicians will work one to one with each child. Magic Care frequently work with seriously ill children and believe that having two magicians visit each child lowers potential distress among performers by giving them the opportunity to talk about their experience together afterwards. Magic Care also provides each child with a small box containing the apparatus required to perform several illusions. This material has been carefully developed to ensure that the illusions are inexpensive to produce, colourful, relatively easy to do, and can be performed in a wide range of situations. The contents of the boxes can be easily tailored to each child's abilities and needs.

Magic Care has published an excellent manual (Greve, 2020). In addition to explaining how to perform several illusions, this manual discusses key psychological factors, including the importance of providing constructive feedback, shifting the spotlight from performer to child, focussing on what each child can do rather than what they can't do, and creating a positive mood. Magic Care also stages workshops for groups, and its manual outlines exercises that can be used in this work. For example, when performing to a group of children, the magician might show the audience a card containing four simple equations. Three of the equations are correct and one is incorrect (e.g. $2 + 2 = 4$; $3 + 6 = 9$; $4 + 2 = 8$; $2 + 1 = 3$). The magician asks the children what they notice, and the majority point out the incorrect equation. After acknowledging that this is the most common response, the magician asks why we all tend to notice what's wrong rather than what's right, and then talks about the importance of compliments over criticisms. I am currently an ambassador for Magic Care, and interview Marlies Greve and Rob van de Kamp later in this chapter.

TEACHING MAGIC TO PRACTITIONERS

Healing of Magic and Magic Therapy™

Early on in his career, illusionist Kevin Spencer was seriously injured in a car accident and had to undergo extensive physical and occupational therapy. He made a full recovery but found the process repetitive and frustrating. As a result, in 1988, Spencer and his wife Cindy created a magic-based programme called Healing of Magic (reorganized and trademarked as Magic Therapy™ in 2018). This initiative involves training health professionals to teach magic to their patients, and Kevin Spencer developed a validated checklist to evaluate how competent therapists are at this task (Yuen & Spencer, 2019). To support this work, the Spencers produced a downloadable manual and an extensive series of online instructional videos that can be used with a variety of patient groups, including those with movement difficulties, and brain and spinal injuries. Kevin Spencer offers courses and workshops on magic therapy, is an Approved Provider of Continuing Education for the American Occupational Therapy Association, and his programme is now used in hospitals and rehabilitation centres across the world.

Side-FX

In 2004, magicians Scott Tokar and Harrison J. Carroll produced an excellent book and DVD on magic for health practitioners (Tokar & Carroll, 2004). They describe tricks and illusions that can be used in various ways, including to help alleviate boredom in waiting rooms, to introduce patients to medical apparatus in a fun way, to reduce anxiety about procedures, and to carry out treatments. For example, to conduct a quick ENT examination with younger patients, practitioners are shown how to place an otoscope speculum on their finger like a thimble, make it disappear, and then use the otoscope to search for it in the child's ear, nose, and throat. Similarly, to introduce medical apparatus in a lighthearted way, they are shown how to make cotton balls magically jump from hand to hand, have a coin magically penetrate through a rubber surgical glove, and to cut and restore the rubber tubing on a stethoscope.

MagicAid

This programme was founded in 2014 by medical students Harrison Pravder and David Elkin at the Renaissance School of

Medicine at Stony Brook University (Elkin & Pravder, 2018), and has since expanded to seven additional medical schools across the United States. MagicAid focuses on training medical students and healthcare professionals to perform magic, with hundreds of pre-clinical students enrolling in this voluntary programme each year. After attending an introductory session, the students participate in small-group training in which they learn basic illusions, and are shown how to interact with patients, comply with hospital protocols, and deliver magic therapy (Pravder et al., 2022). The students then work with both patients and their families in a variety of settings, including paediatric units, paediatric intensive care units, and outpatient centres. These involve students performing several illusions one on one, teaching the child how to perform a trick, and encouraging them to perform for their family, friends, and staff. The scheme aims to help prevent burnout among students, to encourage them to be empathic caregivers, and to provide experience of paediatric care.

Carlo Alfredo Clerici

Clinical psychologist Carlo Alfredo Clerici has recently described how he and his colleagues use magic to support patients at an Italian Paediatric Oncology Unit (Clerici et al., 2021). Part of this work involves practitioners performing magic to aid patient communication. For instance, Clerici describes a psychologist asking an uncommunicative 5-year-old patient whether he had a frog in his stomach, and then using a secret device to produce the sound of a frog each time the child opened his mouth. Magic is also used to help patients to share their thoughts and concerns, and this is illustrated by the case of a 7-year-old child who was upset because he believed that his illness could cause his heart to suddenly stop. The child was a fan of the Harry Potter books and so the psychologist suggested that he may possess magical abilities. The child was given a pen and asked to write the words 'Beauty', 'Joy', 'Serenity', and 'Heart Stopping' on a piece of paper. An illusion was used to reduce the child's anxiety by making the words 'Heart Stopping' disappear.

RESEARCH

Physical Benefits

Green et al. (2013, 2016) had children with hemiplegia complete three movement-related assessments (The Assisting Hand Assessment, The Children's Hand Experience Questionnaire, and The Jebsen-Taylor Test of Hand Function), attend a Breathe magic course (10 six-hour sessions), and then complete the tests a second time and again three months later. The children showed significant improvements on all three assessments.

In a follow-up study, Weinstein et al. (2015) used the same assessments, along with functional brain-imaging scans. The participants again showed improved scoring following the course, and the brain scans indicated increased activation in the affected hemisphere, with around half of the children exhibiting significant increases in white matter integrity in the corpus callosum and corticospinal tract. Schertz et al. (2016) generally replicated these findings and suggested that children with greater severity of brain damage tended to exhibit larger improvements in bilateral hand function, but less change on unimanual function.

Hines et al. (2019) examined the impact of children with hemiplegia participating in a 10-day magic course. Participants completed several assessments before and immediately after the course, and then again three and six months later. In general, participants showed improvements in their affected hand but not in their bimanual ability.

Finally, Spencer et al. (2020) examined how his magic therapy course affected seven children with hemiparesis. A magician showed occupational therapy students how to teach magic tricks to the children, and the therapists then delivered a two-week programme (three days a week, four hours a day). Tests of movement (The Jebsen Hand Function Test, The Children's Hand Experience Questionnaire, and a test of bilateral upper limb motor function) were administered before the intervention, immediately afterwards, and three months later. Participants' scores on all assessments were significantly higher in the three-month follow up.

Psychosocial Benefits

Inspired by Project Magic, occupational therapist Mike Lyons created a similar initiative at hospitals and day therapy centres in Brisbane during the late 1980s. Lyons also conducted what I believe to be the first study to assess the impact of magic on wellbeing (Lyons & Menolotto, 1990). This study took place at an inpatient psychiatric unit and involved people diagnosed with mental health issues. The intervention involved seven weekly sessions in which participants were encouraged to perform simple illusions in a relaxed and supportive atmosphere, and to also practise in their free time. In the final week, they performed a magic show. Learning magic boosted participants' self-esteem and made them more sociable, in part, because it helped them to shift their conversation away from negative topics (e.g. the side effects of medication).

Geens (2005) documented the impact of Project Magic on a paediatric oncology ward in Belgium. Based on a series of case studies, Geens describes how teaching patients magic raised their self-esteem, provided a welcome source of distraction before operations, and helped them to shift their attention away from symptoms.

Inspired by Kevin Spencer's Healing of Magic initiative, Sui and Sui (2007) examined whether patients diagnosed with mental health issues benefited from learning magic. Spencer taught health practitioners a version of the Healing of Magic programme and encouraged them to incorporate magic tricks into their therapy and treatments. Participants completed a measure of life satisfaction (Personal Wellbeing Index) and manual dexterity (Purdue Pegboard) before and after learning the magic, and the post intervention scores were significantly higher. In addition, most participants believed that their memory and concentration had improved, that they had become more confident and were better able to engage in conversation.

Kwong and Cullen (2007) conducted a pilot study into the effects of Healing of Magic on inpatients with an acquired brain injury. Eleven participants attended weekly magic sessions in small groups, and five participants rated their quality of life (EQ-5D Health Questionnaire) and self-esteem (Rosenberg Self-Esteem Scale) before and after the intervention. There were no significant changes. However, only a small sub-set of participants provided the data, and interviews with nine participants revealed that learning magic had helped to break up the day and had made them feel more important.

Hines et al. (2018) explored the psychosocial impact of teaching magic to children with hemiplegia via semi-structured interviews with their parents. First, the children benefited from being around others with similar physical challenges, feeling included, and developing new friendships. Second, the children were motivated by the idea of learning magic and the thought of going to school and being able to do something that the other children couldn't do. Finally, the children showed an increase in self-belief, a willingness to attempt challenging tasks, and the spontaneous use of their affected hand.

Similarly, Fancourt et al. (2020) examined the mechanisms underpinning change in children with hemiplegia during Breathe magic courses. Interviews with children and their parents revealed several benefits, including those associated with reflective motivation (improvements in self-confidence, the development of a 'can do' mindset and increased optimism about the future), social opportunity (forming new friendships due, in part, to being able to do something that other children couldn't do), automatic motivation (increased feelings of pride, independence, and expectations about being able to do something after hard work), and physical capability (being able to complete various tasks, such as getting dressed, having a shower, and making lunch). Parents also noted that the course provided an upbeat topic to talk about with friends and family.

Lee et al. (2022a) examined whether learning magic improved the thinking skills of older individuals exhibiting mild cognitive impairment. Participants either took part in a magic course or were asked to maintain their regular physical and social activities. Before and after questionnaires and tests showed that learning magic resulted in significantly higher general cognitive functioning and faster reaction time. Similarly, Lee et al. (2022b) evaluated whether learning magic reduced depressive symptoms in a group of older adults. Participants were randomly assigned to either a 6-week magic course or a control group in which they maintained their usual activities. Those learning the magic reported significantly lower levels of depressive symptoms.

Reducing Patient Anxiety and Pain

Peretz and Gluck (2005) conducted a study with young children (aged 3–6 years) who were viewed as uncooperative (e.g. refusing to sit in the dentist's chair) either watch some magic or take part in a traditional anxiety-lowering intervention in which they were told what was about to happen and shown a simulated procedure. Those children who had seen the magic sat in the dentist's chair quicker, were more likely to consent to X-rays, and exhibited more cooperative behaviour.

Labrocca and Piacentini (2015) conducted a study with hospitalised children (aged 3–12 years) whose blood samples needed to be collected. Some of the children watched magic during the procedure while the others didn't receive any intervention. The children's self-reported pain ratings revealed that 34% of those who saw the magic reported no pain compared to 12% of those in the other group.

Finally, Pravder et al. (2019) conducted the first randomised study into the therapeutic benefits of magic. Children on a paediatric ward completed a self-report measure of anxiety (The Facial Image Scale, the Venham Picture Test, and/or The Short State-Trait Anxiety Inventory), and either received 15-minutes of MagicAid therapy or no intervention. The children then completed the anxiety measures again, and those who had received the magic intervention completed the measures a third time about an hour later. MagicAid resulted in a significant reduction in anxiety, and this effect was still present after an hour. The children's caregivers also completed the same measures, and those whose children had received MagicAid were significantly less anxious.

Benefits to Medical Practitioners

Pravder et al. (2022) had medical students who had been involved with MagicAid take part in a focus group and/or a survey. The programme resulted in several important benefits, including enhanced communication skills, increased empathy and leadership, better hospital familiarity, and improved psychological health.

PRACTITIONER INTERVIEWS

Marlies Greve and Rob van de Kamp: Magic Care

Magic Care is based in the Netherlands and focuses on teaching magic to children in hospitals and staging workshops for vulnerable groups. I interviewed two people who helped to create the organisation and are still highly involved in its work: President Marlies Greve and Vice-President Rob van de Kamp.

When and How Did Magic Care Start?

Rob: We were originally involved in a project that aimed to improve and promote children's magic. In one of the early meetings of this group, I explained that I was especially interested in using magic to help vulnerable and ill children. Marlies was at the same meeting and she was interested in the same idea. As a result, the two of us got to know one another and decided to create an organisation that focussed on those aims. So, I think the original idea was mine, but Marlies was the one that really had the energy and skills to make it all happen.

Marlies: I am a play therapist and a magician. I have always used magic in my work. It seemed natural to create an organisation that could make a real difference to children's lives. In 2004, Rob and I invited three other magicians (Igor de Kort, Wim van Dokkum, and Rody Boon) over to my house and we founded Magic Care. Our first project involved working with children from Croatia.

What Has Been the Key to Your Success?

Rob: Deep friendship has always sat at the heart of Magic Care. We all love one another and want to help children in need. I think that's important because that kind of positive mindset comes out in our performances. Also, Marlies has always been central to our success because she has an incredible work ethic and an amazing way of interacting with people.

Marlies: I like this interview.

Rob: I am not done yet! Marlies has been a great teacher to all of us and you will see that in all facets of the organisation. She is vital to everything that we do.

Marlies: Thank you. We have made Magic Care together. Early on, there were just a few of us but now there are about 50 magicians involved. It wasn't easy to grow because we felt like a small family. But other magicians heard about our work and they wanted to join us. Once that happened, we took on more of an organising role. At first, about 15 magicians were interested in becoming part of Magic Care and the biggest challenge was to change their mindset. Most magicians enjoy the spotlight and like showing people what they can do. We had to explain the importance of not being the centre of attention and how to put the children first. For some performers that was very strange.

Rob: All the magicians receive two days of training about how to perform with vulnerable children. During this time, we describe the type of children they will see, what they need to do on the wards, how to interact with vulnerable children, and so on. It can be tough, but the rewards are high. We had one very experienced magician who had been performing for most of his life. He said that performing for the children during Magic Care gave him a new and wonderful feeling.

What Is That Feeling?

Rob: It's the feeling that you get from helping others. None of us are paid. We do it to see the children smile and to make them feel proud. The children's parents often become very emotional too because suddenly their child isn't defined by their illness or problems and is instead performing magic.

Marlies: It's so nice because you get a very quick result. It's a very strange thing to see. We have a very positive way of doing magic. A way that makes the child feel safe and accepted. We accept the child and do not ask about their problems. When a child is rude or aggressive, we accept that.

Obviously, we set borders and limitations, but we listen to each child in an active way and find a way of working with them. I have never seen a child that isn't beautiful. There might be something in their behaviour that you don't like, but a child is so much more than their behaviour.

How Do the Magic Care Performances Work?

Rob: We arrange both one-to-one performances and workshops. The one-to-one work involves teaching magic to a single child in a hospital, usually at their bedside. We work closely with hospital staff. They identify children that they think will benefit from seeing and learning magic. We have eye-catching Magic Care trolleys, so that when the magicians walk through the hospital everyone knows who they are. We always arrange for two performers to see each child. This has several advantages. First, sometimes it's stressful for the performers to work with very ill children, and so having two magicians allows them to chat about their feelings with one another afterwards. Second, there are often other family members, such as the child's brother and sisters, in the room and having two magicians allows us to give them some attention too. The performances tend to be much quieter than a regular magic show, and they usually involve one magician performing a trick and the other one explaining it to the child. Typically, we spend around 15 minutes with each child and then leave them with a box of apparatus so that they can practise.

Marlies: The workshops are different. They include a lot of children and can last a couple of hours. One of the key aspects of this work involves encouraging the children to perform and to compliment each other. I have an exercise where we show four equations to people. Three of the equations are correct and one is wrong. I ask everyone in the group what they notice and almost everyone focuses on the equation that is wrong. I then use this to talk about how people tend to criticise others and the importance of complimenting what they can do well.

That's Great. Did You Create That Exercise?

Marlies: Yes and thank you. Then, when each child demonstrates a magic trick, their friends are encouraged to point out what was good about the performance. To help with this, we give each child several cards containing compliments and show them how to use them to deliver positive feedback.

Rob: We also encourage the children to give the compliments in the first person. So, instead of saying 'She did really well', they have to say, 'You did really well'. We have also discovered that the child performing the trick often didn't know what to do when they are given a compliment, and so now we now show them how to look at the person who said something nice and to thank them. This all works because they think that this is how you learn in magic, and they don't realise that the exercise has therapeutic value.

Marlies: We also tell the children that the same idea applies to themselves. Rather than being self-critical, they should compliment themselves on what they can do well. This encourages them to see themselves in a much more positive way, and it stops them thinking 'Oh I can't do that' or 'I am not very good at that'. It's a simple but powerful idea.

Richard Mcdougall: Breathe Magic

Founded in 2010, the Breathe Magic Intensive Therapy Programme teaches magic tricks to young people with hemiplegia to improve their movement and self-confidence. Magician Richard McDougall has been involved with the programme since its inception.

Can You Tell Me How Breathe Started?

David Owen is a barrister and a magician, and he's interested in how magic can promote health. David asked several hospitals if they were interested in the idea and The Evelina London Children's

Hospital invited him in for a chat. He took me along to that first meeting, and the occupational therapists told us about young people with hemiplegia, which is a brain injury that causes paralysis or severe weakness on one side of the body. The children needed to repeat certain actions during therapy, but they often found the exercises repetitive and boring. The therapists demonstrated some of the movements and asked whether magic could be used to make them more meaningful and interesting. We went away, came up with some tricks and returned a few weeks later. The therapists loved what we had done, and we worked together to create a 10-day magic-based intensive therapy programme. We piloted it with a small group of young people, and it worked very well. And that's how it all started.

You've Delivered the Programme Many Times. What Are the Key Learnings?

First, we're not teaching them to be magicians but rather helping them to live a more independent life. Magic is the vehicle. You can't just teach a trick and hope that the children will learn something. Instead, the occupational therapy and the required movements always come first. For example, the children need to be able to use their finger and thumb to pick up objects, and so we might teach a trick using a sponge ball and emphasise the importance of pinching the ball between the finger and thumb. Similarly, stretching out an arm is important so that they can put on a jacket or shirt, and so we might encourage them to hold out apparatus in front of them before they perform a trick. These movements become habit forming, which is what we're looking for.

Second, it's important to find the right magicians. As a performer, you've got to be able to leave your ego at the door. It's not about you or people being amazed by what you can do. You're in the room to help the children and to be part of something bigger. Lots of performers struggle with that and want to be the centre of attention. There was a famous British magician named David Devant and his posters carried a lovely phrase: All done by kindness. That's our mantra. Kindness and compassion are crucial. And the performers must be very good communicators because many of the participants are suffering from mental health issues. I can understand that because it must be very frustrating. If you're 7 years old, it might be OK for your parents to cut up your food, but what about when you're 17 years and you want to go out on a date? But the results are tremendous.

What's Involved in a Typical Programme?

In terms of age, participants range from around 7 to 17 years old. We have one magician at the front, the participants sitting at tables around them and an occupational therapist sitting behind each person. The magician performs the trick and then breaks it down into several steps. They then go through each step, with the participants copying their movements, and the occupational therapists guiding and helping them.

It isn't easy, especially when it comes to putting these actions together and remembering the correct sequence. For example, one classic magic trick involves three balls appearing and disappearing under three cups. When you perform it, you've got to remember the set-up, where the balls are, the correct order of the actions, and so on. But amazingly, you get to a point where you see the whole class doing it correctly and that's very rewarding.

We grade every trick in terms of difficulty. So, with something like the jumping band trick, you can grade whether a child can pick the band up in their affected hand, place it over their two fingers, carry out the secret move, and so on. Then can they do it using their other hand? All the tricks are graded, and we move from simple tricks to more challenging ones across the 10 days. We want to teach the participants to perform the tricks well because we have a duty of care to protect them socially. There's nothing worse than a child performing a trick at school and their friends figuring it out. That would do more harm than good.

And the Course Builds to a Final Show?

Yes. That's vital. Sometimes we have as many as 150 people in the audience, including parents, health professionals, friends, and so on. It's in a proper theatre, so the participants have to learn how to be on a stage with lighting, how to use sound cues, and so on.

We work on their performance skills from day one, starting with something as simple as having them stand up at the front of the room and saying their name.

How Does the Programme Change People?

It's amazing to see what young people can achieve by the end of the course. For example, we had one person who was going to University and had never held a knife and fork. By the end of the programme, they were cutting their own food and were far more confident. And it's not just about movement. When it comes to confidence, magic is like rocket fuel. It really boosts their confidence and expectations about what they can do in other areas of their life. I've seen some children move up in class because they suddenly feel more confident to read and others take part in school plays. A few weeks ago, a 15-year-old girl arrived wearing a tee-shirt that had three simple words on it: Actually, I can. I was like, wow. That's the attitude!

How Much of That Is To Do with Them Being Able to Accomplish Something That Looks Impossible?

That's a very good question. I think it's vital. We perform a magic trick that looks completely impossible, and then break the trick into steps, and encourage them to work hard and master each of these steps. They then apply that mindset to other aspects of their lives, such as tying their shoelaces or whatever. They start to believe that maybe they can achieve these tasks if they break them down into small steps, work hard, and don't give up. They generate that positive mindset themselves. That's the key.

What Role Do the Parents Play During the Programme?

They are not present when we teach magic. They drop the children off in the morning and only come back when it's time to pick them up. During the programme, we try to have participants be as independent as possible, and often we encourage the parents to adopt the same attitude. I can see why that's difficult. For example, if you're rushing out of the house in the morning, it's easy to tie a child's shoelaces for them or whatever. But we encourage them to step back and to let their child try to do more things for themselves. It often makes a real difference. One reward for me is seeing the parents at the end of the programme. Often, they are very emotional because of the effect that is has on their lives. Sometimes it's as simple as the family having had their first Sunday lunch where they've sat down together and their child has cut up their own food.

Can You Tell Me More About How This Work Makes You Feel?

For me, it feels far, far, more meaningful than a regular performance. We have lots of busy professional magicians involved in the programme, and I suspect that they will all tell you that it's the best thing they do. By far the best thing. Can you imagine seeing a child who had their hand closed all their life, suddenly be able to open their hand? And to see the difference that that makes to their life? And to know that you played a role in making that happen? It's a wonderful feeling. It has to be. It's transformative. It really is.

SUMMARY

The chapter has explored the many ways in which magic can be used within a medical setting. Much of this work involves teaching magic to patients with movement issues to make repetitive actions more meaningful and enjoyable. Additional work has examined how learning magic boosts patients' self-esteem, in part, because it emphasises strengths over weaknesses and results in them being able to do something that others cannot do. Socially, performing magic for others offers a novel way of connecting with friends, family, and medical staff, and provides patients with a new interest and a positive topic of conversation. On a more conceptual level, magic makes the impossible seem possible and so encourages patients to have hope and to believe that they can recover. Finally, practitioners can use magic to reduce patient's pain and anxiety, to introduce medical apparatus in a fun way, and to help to carry out some procedures and treatments.

3

CONJURING UP LIFE SKILLS

Applied Magic has helped to build a range of key life skills, including confidence, lateral thinking, preparedness, and resilience. This work has involved a variety of individuals, including people with learning differences and psychological conditions, those who are marginalised within society, and broad groups of children and adults. This chapter reviews each of these areas.

LEARNING DIFFERENCES AND PSYCHOLOGICAL CONDITIONS

The Magic Kids

In the early 1980s, American teacher Sadie Broome created The Magic Kids (Broome, 1995). This programme aims to help school children (aged 8–12 years old) with behavioural and emotional challenges, and involves them attending several magic lessons and staging a show for younger pupils. Broome recommends developing two identical shows with two groups of children, so that if a child is unable or unwilling to perform in the show, the corresponding person from the other group can step into the role and the show can still go ahead. During the first lesson, the children take an oath of secrecy. Each child then decides whether they want to be a performer, a technician, a prop maker, or an audience member. The group then works together, selecting illusions, building apparatus, creating presentations, and rehearsing. These activities present an opportunity to emphasise the importance of collaboration, trusting one another, providing positive feedback, and creating something for others to enjoy. In addition, The Magic Kids offers the children a new and positive sense of identity and belonging.

Hocus Focus™

In 2009, American magician Kevin Spencer built upon the success of his Magic Therapy programme (see Chapter Two) to create Hocus Focus™. This magic course aims to support students who have learning differences, behavioural challenges, and psychological conditions. Spencer developed the content in collaboration with educational practitioners, and the lessons are designed to promote key cognitive skills, including planning, sequencing, organisation, concentration, and memory. The course is flexible and can be taught one-on-one or to groups. Those interested in teaching Hocus Focus™ can purchase various online resources, including lesson plans (aligned with America's National and Common Core State Standards of Learning), a teaching manual, and an instructional video. Spencer et al. (2019) developed and validated a scale for measuring the expertise of coaches delivering this material, and O'Rourke et al. (2018) created a self-report instrument to measure student growth in cognition, motor skills, communication, social skills, and creativity (assessing, for example, whether the student remembers the correct sequence of events, captures the audience's interest, etc.).

Child Counselling

Some child counsellors and educators perform and teach magic to help their clients and students. Much of this work involves using illusions to convey positive messages, including the importance of making friends, being kind, talking about emotions, dealing with anger, and avoiding drug and alcohol misuse (Bowman, 1986, 2004; Goodman & Furman, 1981; Spruill & Poidevant, 1993). For example, Bowman (2004) uses the Book of Spells (see Chapter

One) to illustrate the importance of sharing emotions. In this presentation, the performer shows that a notebook contains black and white illustrations, lists several colours, and asks the child what emotion they associate with each colour. The performer then tells the child to pretend to throw these colours towards the book, shows that it's now full of colourful illustrations and discusses how feelings enrich people's lives. In another example, the performer uses Through a Postcard (see Chapter One) to illustrate how seemingly impossible problems can have surprisingly simple solutions. Bowman (2004) also presents practical advice about how to run a school-based magic club, including providing forms for parental consent and membership, a checklist for evaluating presentations (e.g. whether the child stood up straight, looked at the audience, spoke clearly, etc.), and a certificate of completion.

Other work involves using magic to increase rapport and to aid diagnosis.

In an early monograph, Howard (1977, as cited in Stehouwer, 1983) outlines ways in which magic can be used with children who are reluctant to engage with the counsellor. For example, he suggests that counsellors could say that they are going to practise some magic, explain that no one has ever figured out the secret to the trick and then perform an illusion that isn't especially fooling. Howard says that children are often eager to explain that they have worked out the solution and that this interaction can then act as a catalyst for more meaningful engagement.

Stehouwer (1983) explores how performing magic motivates children to attend future sessions and how teaching parents to perform simple illusions can help them to interact with their family. Stehouwer also notes how magic goes against the ethos of having an honest relationship with clients and so advises counsellors to avoid overusing the word 'trick' and being open to explaining how their illusions work.

Some writers (e.g. Gilroy, 1998) have also suggested that monitoring a child's reaction to magic might help provide an insight into whether they might have attentional issues (unable to concentrate on the performance), low impulse control (reaching for apparatus) or poor emotional regulation (becoming angry when the performer refuses to reveal the secret of the illusion).

INDIVIDUALS MARGINALISED WITHIN SOCIETY

Several Applied Magic programmes aim to help individuals who are marginalised in society, including those affected by poverty, social exclusion, violence, unemployment, and discrimination.

The College of Magic

The College of Magic was founded in South Africa by magician David Gore in 1980. For more than 40 years, it has taught magic to hundreds of students, with many attendees coming from disadvantaged backgrounds. The College currently offers two introductory courses (aimed at children aged 10–13 and 14–17 years) that combine magic with allied skills such as mime, clowning, puppetry, juggling, and ventriloquism. Senior students also receive training in theatrical and technical skills including sound, lighting, and filmmaking. Each of the hour-long weekly sessions takes place on an extramural basis and involves voluntary teaching staff helping students to develop eight Star Qualities (Honesty, Respect, Responsibility, Initiative, Excellence, Empathy, Humility, and Wonder). The courses offer multiple performing opportunities and aim to help students to develop key psychological skills, including confidence, enthusiasm, initiative, responsibility, self-discipline, determination, and passion. Graduating students can take further courses that help them to gain additional expertise in specific areas of their choice with many spending several years training at the College. The College is especially keen to provide students from disadvantaged backgrounds with the opportunity to enrol in the courses and to celebrate South Africa's cultural diversity. These students are selected with the assistance of local schools and community leaders, and the experience aims to improve their academic performance, to encourage them to move away from illegal activities, to develop their leadership abilities, and to be proud of their community. Importantly, the College also helps students to become economically independent by encouraging them to seek out paid performing opportunities at restaurants, parties, and special events. For a detailed discussion about this work, see my interview with David Gore and Marian Williamson later in this chapter.

Magic Care

In the Netherlands, Magic Care (see Chapter Two) helps refugees and individuals from other marginalised groups. Much of this work involves magicians holding workshops for groups of children (aged 8–15 years old). Most recently, this has involved working with refugees displaced by the war in Ukraine. As noted previously, Magic Care has pioneered the creation of cost-effective boxes containing the apparatus needed to perform magic and demonstrated the agility of this approach by quickly translating instructions in order to produce bespoke boxes for use in this work.

My Magic Hands

Chapter Two described how My Magic Hands helps children in Canadian hospitals. This programme also delivers magic courses to communities from poor, inner-city areas. These programmes tend to involve adult and teenage volunteers helping younger children with after-school activities under the direction of a magician. This type of mentoring scheme encourages community participation, allows for one-to-one support, provides participants with a positive peer model, and gives the volunteers valuable work experience. My Magic Hands has also teamed up with a charitable foundation that supports newcomers to Canada. In this instance, the newcomers acted as the volunteers and supported younger children learning magic. This novel approach helped to ensure that the newcomers were placed in an empowering role. Many of these programmes involve participants staging a magic show for their friends and family, and this helps to structure the programme, provides participants with a concrete goal, and extends community reach. The work aims to help participants grow in confidence, and to view both themselves and their communities in a more positive and productive way. For more information about this work, see my interview with Julie Eng at the end of this chapter.

Edinburgh International Magic Festival

Svetlana McMahon (Edinburgh International Magic Festival) and I have staged illusion-based photography exhibitions with two charities. One of the charities supports young carers from areas of high deprivation whilst the other helps to combat homelessness among young people. These projects involve working with young carers or unhoused young people to create images based on various optical illusions, such as using perspective to make a person appear to be much smaller than they are. The resulting images are then displayed in exhibitions that present and explain the illusions. This experience offers participants an opportunity to demonstrate their creativity and imagination, and to help increase their confidence and social networks. Each exhibition is staged across two locations, with one location presenting the images and the other containing videos of the participants describing their lives and explaining how the illusions were created. Participants often invite their friends and family to the exhibition, and act as visitor guides.

Magicians Without Borders

This initiative was founded by Tom Verner and his wife Janet Fredericks in 2002. Their mission is to 'use the art of magic to entertain, educate and empower forgotten children around the world, primarily refugee and orphan children'. They have travelled to more than 40 countries, performing in refugee camps, orphanages, hospitals, and even abandoned buildings. Magicians Without Borders also has seven Sorcerer's Apprentice Educational Programmes around the world. These programmes are directed by a local magician in collaboration with a partner organisation. They teach adolescents magic to help to promote several key skills, including confidence, focus, discipline, and self-esteem. Magicians Without Borders has discovered that learning, practising, and performing magic awakens a sense of hope and helps to demonstrate how a once unimagined life might be possible. The organisation has a Scholarship Fund that helps to make these dreams a reality. For more information about this initiative, see my interview with Tom Verner later in this chapter.

Magic for Smiles

Jamie Balfour-Paul founded the charity Magic for Smiles and has used magic to provide psychosocial support to young, traumatised, refugees in Jordan, Turkey, Lebanon, and Britain. Balfour-Paul performs and teaches magic to help lower distress and to enhance wellbeing, and has collaborated with several non-government organisations and community-based groups.

Streets of Growth and Prison Work

In 2001, youth worker and magician Darren Way co-founded Streets of Growth, a charity that works in one of London's most socio-economically deprived boroughs to prevent young adults from becoming involved in gang violence and criminality (Wiseman et al., 2022). Way uses magic to establish rapport with 'harder to reach' young adults and to begin to identify gang hierarchies. This intervention work involves encouraging young adults to attend his leadership development centre by showing them some close-up magic on the street and then offering to train them in magic at his centre. Way has found that these types of approaches are especially effective with young adults who feel insecure and are attracted to the idea of knowing something that other people don't know. However, Way also believes that although magic can play a beneficial role in establishing contact and building rapport, real progress only comes from systemic changes associated with providing opportunities for education and employment, building safer communities, dealing with past trauma, and equipping people to move away from problematic circumstances.

Finally, magician and counsellor Gareth Foreman has extensive experience working in custodial settings and prisoner rehabilitation, and has developed and delivered magic workshops that aim to reduce re-offending. An initial part of these workshops involves performing magic for participants and having them work together to figure out how the illusions were achieved. After generating lots of ideas, participants are encouraged to think about how the same ideas might be used to solve issues in their own life. According to Foreman, many of the participants have become involved in crime because it provides instant gratification, and that slowly working out the secrets to the illusions encourages them to develop patience and perseverance. In addition, the workshops enhance participants' problem-solving skills by emphasising that there are different ways of looking at a problem and that challenging issues can often have surprisingly simple solutions. Participants also perform magic to one another, and Foreman believes that this is helpful because it involves them adopting various roles, including those of a magician, a helper, and an audience member. This helps to build their self-confidence and encourages perspective-taking, trust, and empathy.

CHILDREN AND ADULTS

Several initiatives use magic to encourage life skills among more general cohorts of children and adults, although it's likely that some of the individuals taking part have the learning differences and psychological conditions described earlier in this chapter.

Discover Magic

Discover Magic aims to help teach important life skills to children (Johnston, 2016). Participants are taught bespoke illusions that emphasise respect, preparedness, enthusiasm, confidence, humility, creativity, authenticity, and altruism. Participants receive a file of secret instructions, the apparatus required to perform the magic, and access to online videos. At the end of the course, they are also given a graduation certificate and a magic wand. Magicians purchase a licence to present Discover Magic in their local community, with the organisers aiming to ensure that a limited number of licences are granted in any given area. Each magician is provided with a comprehensive manual explaining how to find clients and present the course in a variety of settings, including camps, schools, and libraries. The course is highly flexible, allowing magicians to alter the curriculum to fit their personality and circumstances.

Growth Mindset

Several projects use magic to encourage a growth mindset (a belief that people can change through hard work and dedication).

In one initiative, I teamed up with highly experienced children's entertainer David Kaye (aka Silly Billy) to devise presentations that magicians can use to encourage various life skills in younger audiences (Wiseman & Kaye, 2020). This work is based on observational learning, wherein children imitate the behaviour of those around them. We created three presentations in which the performer exhibits various positive qualities. For example, when performing a version of the Book of Spells, the performer shows the blank notebook and explains that they are struggling to make drawings magically appear. Next, they ask the children to help by pretending to hold a magic black crayon and by scribbling in the air. The pages of the book remain blank, and the performer encourages the children to keep trying and to work together. Eventually, the black and white drawings magically appear in the book and the performer asks everyone if they would like to try something even harder. The children are asked to rub their fingers on a piece of coloured clothing and to throw the colour at the book. Finally, the performer shows that the book now contains lots of colourful drawings. This presentation encourages children to tackle difficult challenges, to work together, and to persevere in the face of adversity. In the other presentations, the children discover the importance of emotional regulation and to learn techniques for dealing with sadness and anger.

In addition, I worked with Kevin Quantum and Svetlana McMahon (The Edinburgh International Magic Festival) and children's entertainer Magic Gareth to produce a family magic show entitled *You Are Magic*. During the show, members of the audience become the stars of the show and perform several seemingly impossible feats, including large illusions, mind reading and escapology. The show encourages the audience to discover their potential, to support one another and to use their imagination. To highlight this message, most of the apparatus is created from cardboard boxes and other everyday objects.

Magic Gareth (2021) has written a book that shows children how to make a dog out of a modelling balloon and encourages them to persevere with difficult tasks. Similarly, Amy Kimlat's (2022) book, *Hocus Pocus Practice Focus*, aims to attract more girls into magic and emphasises the importance of hard work and study.

Finally, I recently teamed up with the College of Magic to produce a book entitled *Everybody's Magic*. This features students from the College teaching readers how to perform illusions, describes the inspirational life stories of people who dedicated their lives to the art of magic, and outlines important life lessons. This book aims to promote diversity and to celebrate master magicians who tend not to appear in beginners' books on magic.

Abracademy

At an adult level, London-based Abracademy delivers magic workshops that encourage team building and aim to help organisations tackle various issues, including those associated with change management, communication, and leadership. By watching and performing magic, participants develop several skills that are helpful in the workplace, including increased self-confidence (removing limiting beliefs and unlocking hidden talents), a more open mindset (achieving the impossible), enhanced creativity (identifying assumptions and looking at an issue from different perspectives), and greater connectedness (instilling a sense of belonging and collaborating with colleagues).

RESEARCH

Self-Confidence and Self-Esteem

Ezell and Klein-Ezell (2003) conducted a study with school children (aged 5–16 years old) who had behavioural issues and learning differences. Participants completed a measure of self-esteem (a subscale of the Student Self-Concept Scale) before and after learning several illusions over the course of a semester. The children were shown how to cope with the challenges that might arise during a performance and role-played how to respond when spectators asked them to expose the secret. They also eventually performed for younger pupils and their peers. The children's self-esteem scores were significantly higher after learning magic, with the researchers ascribing this to them developing coping skills and being able to do something that other people couldn't do.

Levin (2007) worked with nine children and students who had exhibited poor conduct in school or had been diagnosed with mental health issues. Many of them had a history of sexual abuse, poor family functioning, and substance abuse. Six of them (aged 6–18 years) completed a measure of self-esteem (Rosenberg's Self-Esteem Scale) before and after learning to perform magic during six one-hour weekly sessions. The authors didn't report any statistical analyses but noted that the post intervention scores were generally higher. The children also exhibited behavioural improvements, including a 65% decrease in interpersonal boundary violations and a 62% decrease in 'time-outs'.

Yuen et al. (2021) had six children diagnosed with Attention Deficit Hyperactivity Disorder (aged 8–14 years) complete a measure of self-esteem (Rosenberg Self-Esteem Scale) before and after attending a four-week online magic course (three days a week, an hour a day). Their scores were significantly higher after learning the magic tricks. In a similar study, Spencer et al. (2022) reported that 16 autistic children (aged 8–15 years) attending the same virtual camp showed increased scoring on measures of self-esteem (Rosenberg Self-Esteem) and social skills (Social Skills Improvement System).

Cognition, Connectedness, and Mood

Spencer (2012) examined whether his Hocus Focus™ programme encourages growth in cognition and positive affect. The evaluation took place in 3 schools, involved 9 teachers and more than 70 students (aged 14–21 years). Some of the students had learning differences, and others were diagnosed with mental health issues. Observation checklists, interviews, and surveys revealed that the teachers believed that the intervention had various benefits, including encouraging engagement, emphasising the importance of following sequential steps, helping to cope with the frustrations of learning a task, and highlighting how to provide others with constructive feedback.

Bonete et al. (2021) had 11 children (aged 8–12 years) diagnosed with Attention Deficit Hyperactivity Disorder participate in 10 magic-based training sessions in which the magic became more challenging as the course progressed. Several cognitive measures were completed at three time periods (before the sessions, immediately afterwards, and three months later), including the Five Digits Test (processing speed, inhibition, cognitive flexibility), the D2 Test of Attention (sustained attention, selective attention, degree of impulsivity), subtests of the Wechsler Intelligence Scale (processing speed, short-term memory, working memory), and the Battery of Neuropsychological Assessment for Executive Function (phonological fluency, semantic fluency, mental flexibility, thought organisation, sequencing, prospective memory). Overall, the participants showed improvements in processing speed, sustained attention, thought organisation, sequencing, working memory, concentration, and cognitive flexibility.

Bagienski (2016) had one group of undergraduates learn magic and another acquire rapport building skills. Each week participants performed the illusions or used the techniques, and then completed daily ratings about their mood and how successful they had been. Contrary to the hypothesis, there were no significant differences between the groups.

Bagienski and Kuhn (2022) had one group of undergraduates complete a magic workshop and another take a mindfulness course. Participants completed measures of self-esteem (Self-Perception Profile for College Students), closeness to others (Inclusion of Other in Self Scale), sense of community (Perceived Cohesion Scale), and wellbeing (general happiness and the Depression, Anxiety, and Stress Scale). These measures were completed before the intervention, immediately afterwards, and one-month later. Both interventions increased scores on the measures, but there was no difference between the groups. Participants also rated the degree to which they thought that the intervention had changed their self-esteem, closeness, sense of community and wellbeing. Those learning magic believed that they had experienced greater levels of improvement, with the authors arguing that this could be due to some of these concepts being made more salient in the magic workshops.

Bagienski et al. (2022) had undergraduates fill out a questionnaire about the degree to which they think that they can achieve future goals (self-efficacy: The Pearlin Mastery scale) and describe the steps that they would take to solve common problems, such as making new friends at university (The Means-Ends Problem-Solving Task). They were then taught some simple magic and completed the measures again. Participants' self-efficacy scores increased, with their difficulty and confidence ratings suggesting that this was because learning the illusion was easier than they had anticipated. There was no change in the student's scores on the problem-solving task. Qualitative analyses suggested that learning the illusion yielded various benefits, including helping participants to develop a more optimistic mindset.

Creativity

I have examined whether learning to perform magic causes children to think more creatively (Wiseman, Wiles et al., 2021). A group of 60 school children (aged 10–11 years) first completed a standard test of creativity that involves listing as many unusual ways of using everyday objects as possible (The Alternative Uses Test). Some of the children were then shown how to perform some simple magic whilst the others were taught how to make an illusion-based perspective drawing. Finally, the children completed the creativity test a second time. Learning the magic resulted in greater increases in creativity, and this might be due to the children watching a seemingly impossible event and/or finding out the lateral solution to the trick.

PRACTITIONER INTERVIEWS

Julie Eng: My Magic Hands

Canadian magician Julie Eng is the executive director of Magicana, an organisation dedicated to furthering the art of conjuring. Julie has created My Magic Hands, a structured but flexible wellbeing programme that has been delivered in a wide variety of contexts.

How Did My Magic Hands Begin?

I started the project when I moved to Toronto from the west coast of Canada. I had previously taught a few magic classes, and wondered if magic could be used to promote participants' physical and psychological health. Magicana is based in Toronto, and magician David Ben is also involved with the organisation. David was interested in the idea and challenged me to create a structured programme that was grounded in educational principles. Thanks to government funding, we developed a course that runs between six and eight weeks. The sessions were designed to build upon one another and so there is a genuine sense of learning and progress.

I Know the Programme Involves Magicians, Coaches, and Participants. Can You Tell Me More About These Roles?

Sure! My Magic Hands is delivered to large groups of participants rather than to individuals. A magician acts as the instructor and is supported by coaches. For instance, in a hospital setting, we have had a magician teach children with brain injuries, with occupational therapists acting as the coaches. In our community work, magicians have worked with students from inner-city and at-risk communities, with high-school volunteers as coaches. Before the course begins, I arrange an orientation for the coaches and explain that they are not expected to teach the magic, but rather to support participants by helping them to learn the trick, to ask questions, and so on. It's nice because the coaches and participants learn together. Each coach wants to help their participant, and each participant wants to make their coach proud. That dynamic is empowering because there's an evenness to the learning. Magic is a great leveller. Participants have different levels of ability and experience when it comes to singing and dancing, but almost none of them have tried magic before.

How Is My Magic Hands Structured?

I start by telling the children that we are going to put on a show at the end of the programme. That often freaks them out and some of them think that it's impossible! And that is the point: to show that with planning and practise, anything becomes possible. I calm everyone down and explain how we're going to work together to learn the tricks and to create the show.

In the first session, they take and sign an oath of secrecy. They love the idea of being initiated into the magic community and of carrying on this important tradition. Then we start to learn some tricks. The first few tricks are relatively easy because I want everyone to enjoy some initial success. As the course progresses, the material becomes more challenging. We encourage everyone to work hard, and we give them a booklet that contains tips and hints, including a chart to tick off how many times they have practiced. There are many key skills threaded through the programme, including how to cope if a trick goes wrong (building planning skills), treating spectators with respect (learning social skills), how to create a script (stimulating creative thinking), how to move on stage (building self-awareness and self-confidence), and so on.

There are also opportunities to perform during the sessions. Besides getting used to being in front of people, the students watch each other and are encouraged to reflect on what does, and doesn't, work. A key part of this involves showing them how to constructively criticise themselves and others. Over time, they bond together and form a close community. The young adults from the inner-city often struggle with trust and so it's especially nice to see them come together like that.

How Do You Build Up to the Final Show?

We put the show together, and then we have a technical and dress rehearsal. The tech helps us to figure out the apparatus that each participant needs, which side they enter the stage from, and so on. During the dress rehearsal, the participants go through the show wearing their costumes, and so this is an opportunity to make sure that the capes don't slip off their shoulders, that the hats don't cover their eyes, etc. Before the dress rehearsal, I make a big speech and remind them how hard they have worked. This is also a good time to explain that they are the stars, but that the show is about them and the audience having a good time.

In many instances, the final performance is for a large group, sometimes up to 150 people, of friends, family, and peers. The lead magician emcees the show and performs between the acts. I really want the participants to succeed, so when I emcee, I watch them like a hawk. But because the children are so well prepared, the tricks go well, and very, very, rarely do I step in to assist. The participants' families aren't directly involved with the sessions, so the show is a big surprise. Each performance normally gets a huge ovation. And, it's not gratuitous because the participants have earned it. Children know when a reaction is fake and when it's real. I am always very proud of them, and it's a big boost to their self-esteem and confidence.

Can You Tell Me More About the Inner-City Work?

Many of the participants from these communities are vulnerable. They face tough situations, and sometimes haven't eaten properly and have their heads on the table because they are so tired. Obviously, it's important that our coaches are properly screened and understand the importance of child safety. Magicana isn't set up to carry out that work, and so we partner with recreation centres in these areas, and seek out their volunteers to be the coaches. This arrangement is great because the centres have a vetted volunteer pool, and have a clear protocol for child safety. Also, the kids often know these volunteers and already have a positive relationship with them. It's also great for the volunteers. In Canada, high-school students are encouraged to volunteer in the community, and becoming one of our coaches provides them with an opportunity to be a positive role model and to make a real difference. In one inner-city project, our coaches were drawn from a group of girls attending a private school in a wealthier area of the city. The girls were 15 to 17 years old and the participants were about 11 years old. It was a huge success. Everyone bonded and sometimes the kids taught the girls how to perform the magic – which they found very empowering. That felt like real magic.

And How About the Hospital Work?

The hospital work mostly involves kids recovering from brain injuries. The children see My Magic Hands as a recreational activity rather than therapy. When an occupational therapist asks them to stack cups, or to try to do up their buttons, they are often resistant. But if we show them how to make a knot magically appear on a rope, they will repeat the movements over and over.

It's amazing to see the kids achieve something that they couldn't do before the programme. For instance, a few years ago, we worked with a nonverbal 6-year-old girl who was paralysed on one side of her body. We encourage the kids to take a bow at the end of their act. We teach them to put one hand in front of them, one hand behind them, and to bend forward at the waist. This little girl struggled with the second part because of her paralysis, but she could bring one hand in front and bow. During the dress rehearsal, she completes her trick and lifts one hand in front, so we start to applaud. She then lifts the *other* hand, the one she hasn't moved since her injury, and places it behind her to complete her bow. The whole room was in tears, and her mother was speechless. I saw this little girl again about a year later and, wow, she was a real chatterbox. That's why I do this work. I see mini miracles like that all the time.

Tom Verner: Magicians Without Borders

Tom Verner is an American psychotherapist, magician, and psychologist. In 2002, he co-founded Magicians Without Borders with his wife Janet. This organisation uses magic to 'entertain, educate and empower forgotten children around the world' and focuses primarily on refugee and orphan children.

How Did You Get into Magic?

Wellbeing and magic came into my life simultaneously. In the early 1970s, I was working as a counsellor in a Drug and Alcohol

Rehabilitation Hospital, and I met a magician who was a recovering heroin addict. I begged him to teach me some magic tricks, but he always refused. Eventually, he was assigned to me as a patient, and we met for an hour each week. At our first meeting, he said, 'Fifty minutes of this session are mine and ten minutes are yours', and for the next two years, he spent those 10 minutes teaching me some great tricks. And that's how I got into magic!

Was Magicians Without Borders Created Around That Time?

No, it was much, much later. I was awarded my PhD in psychology and began working at the State University of New York at New Paltz. I was also teaching psychology to some of the inmates in a local maximum-security prison and occasionally performed magic for them. Then I was invited to participate in a meditative retreat in Poland and I wanted to visit other places in the region. I was prepared to travel about 200 miles from Krakow, and so I took a compass and drew a circle on a map. I had my radio playing in the background, and there was an item about the war in Kosovo. Just as the presenter said the word 'Pristina', which is the capital of Kosovo, my compass landed on the city. Being a Jungian, I take co-incidences seriously, and so I thought about going to Kosovo to perform. I contacted the person organising the retreat and asked if she knew anybody around Kosovo. Amazingly, her friend was working with refugees there and I was eventually put in touch with someone who worked with the United Nations High Commission for Refugees in Kosovo. It all worked out well, and I was invited to perform several shows there.

When I was in Kosovo, my UN driver took me to perform in a village. After the show, a Roma woman came up and handed me a gold coin. She had seen me magically multiply objects during the show and wanted me to make her money grow. Then two Roma men asked me if I could make visas appear. That night, I realised two things. First, magic is a universal language. None of these people spoke English, and I didn't speak Roma or Serbo-Croatian, but we all spoke magic. Second, I thought about a comment once made by the great magician and escapologist Harry Houdini. He was a refugee from Hungary and said that when he did magic for people, especially individuals in difficult circumstances, it not only amazed and amused but also awakened hope and helped them to believe that the impossible might be possible. That was the moment that the idea for Magicians Without Borders was born.

A few months later, I went to my Head of Department at the University and I asked to take a year off to go around the world performing magic in refugee camps. Well, that leave of absence has now gone on for 21 years!

How Did Your Work Develop?

A UN photographer included several pictures of my show in a book about the refugees in Kosovo. Because of that, we became friends, and I told her about wanting to travel around the world doing magic for refugees. I also said that we especially wanted to go to Ethiopia. One of her colleagues coordinated UN projects on the Horn of Africa, and eventually we met a wonderful guy who was the public information officer for the UN High Commission for Refugees in Ethiopia. War and violence in the region had produced four and a half million refugees, and we staged several shows there.

The people working for the UN Commission for Refugees in one place are usually in post for a few years and are then sent to another region. Often, they would see us in one place and then invite us to their new posting. After a while, we were regularly receiving invitations to perform in lots of countries.

What Are the Difficulties with Doing this Kind of Work?

We've done hundreds of shows in many refugee camps and overall had very positive experiences. One issue is that in some places, like Sudan, some people believe that real magic can be used to heal and harm. Early on, when we were performing in Sudanese refugee camps, someone from the UN told us that some spectators were scared by magic and so we had to be careful. Sometimes the answer was to have community leaders explain to the group that we were performing tricks.

The only violence we ever ran into also happened to be in Sudan. A military group had abducted thousands of children, and we went to entertain some of the kids who had been rescued. We were performing in this amazing mango grove, and there was a group of soldiers there. A couple of their friends had been recently killed in the fighting, and they were sad, angry, and drunk. I'm on the back of the truck doing a magic show for the kids and my driver said the drunk soldiers thought that I was doing real miracles and was going to abduct the children. At one point, the leader picks up his AK-47, and he's about to fire at me. My driver quickly pushed me down onto the bed of the truck, then jumped into the driver's seat and sped away.

How Do Your Shows Help People?

Our mission is to use magic to entertain, educate, and empower. Our shows are like a little pebble being thrown into a pond. It causes lots of little ripples that sometimes have a big effect.

I think that we can also help to bring people together. For instance, a few years ago, we did some shows at Sudanese refugee camps and had dinner with one of the Sudanese elders. He explained that although people on the camp laughed and told stories to their family and friends, our show was the first time that the community had joined together and laughed together. At the time, there were two tribes in the camp, and they had very little to do with one another. When they did meet, violence would often break out. The elder explained that people from both tribes were at our show, and that everyone was having a good time.

Another time we were in Iran and an Afghan elder asked us what kind of space we would like for our performance. I said that an inside space would be good for focus and he explained that the only inside space was the mosque, but that he would be honoured to have us perform there. We did two shows, one for 500 girls and then one for 500 boys. Afterwards, the elder explained that he had been in the camp for 17 years and that we were the first entertainers to perform there. He said that the international relief agencies took wonderful care of them and provided food, shelter, and clothing, but that we fed the minds and imaginations of the children and they would be talking about our show for months.

Can You Tell Me About Your Sorcerer's Apprentice Programme?

Magicians Without Borders now encourages children to learn, practice, and perform magic during our Sorcerer's Apprentice programmes. We run six of these courses around the world, in Colombia, Costa Rica, El Salvador, South Africa, and two in India. They are great because we quickly begin to see an increase in the children's confidence, focus, discipline, and self-esteem. Also, on some profound level that I don't fully understand, it awakens the sense of hope that Houdini spoke about.

Magic feeds children's minds and imaginations and awakens their dreams and aspirations. Let me give you a concrete example. I remember one young girl on a Sorcerer's Apprentice programme in El Salvador. She was making a very small amount of money selling beans in the market with her mother, but told us that she wanted to be a nurse. The nursing school wasn't far from the market, and the nurses would walk past in their beautiful white starched uniforms. At the time, it seemed impossible that this young girl could achieve her ambition. However, she had hope and persevered and now works as a geriatric nurse. She makes more money in one day than she did working for two months in the market, and she's bought her mother a house. She is also a pebble in the pond because she has inspired her sister to go to college. I can tell you many stories like that. Encouraging children to learn, practice, and perform magic awakens hope and helps them to believe that the seemingly impossible might one day be possible.

David Gore and Marian Williamson: The College of Magic

The College of Magic was founded by David Gore. The College is based in Cape Town, and both David and educator Marian Williamson have played key roles in ensuring the success of the initiative. Over a hundred students are enroled at the College each year, with many of them coming from disadvantaged backgrounds.

When and How Did the College Start?

David: My great grandfather worked as a puppeteer and had brought Punch and Judy figures from Britain to South Africa. My father often helped with the shows and so there was a little bit of performance in our family. As a youngster, I performed magic during my high-school years here in Cape Town, and I met lots of young people who wanted to learn magic. There were very few books about magic available in libraries, and so a colleague and I decided to open the College of Magic. That was in 1980, when I was 19 years old. Local journalists wrote some articles about the College and we had 34 students enroled. That's how it all started.

Marian: Also, before he started the College, David used to have underprivileged youngsters visit his home and perform acrobatics, and so on. And he taught them magic too.

David: Yes. I was from what would be classed as a liberal family at the time. Apartheid was operating in South Africa, and so everything was very restricted. I was brought up in a household that encouraged reaching out and helping. We wanted to see a more inclusive society and so we would invite these youngsters over. Those became some of the first students at the College.

What's the Secret of the College's Continued Success?

David: I think diversity is vital. From day one, we involved people from all racial and socioeconomic groups. During apartheid, our students were having to travel in separate train carriages, and so on. Having a place where everyone could come together was hugely important. That was back in the 1980s, but even now that sense of inclusivity is important and relevant.

Marian: Yes, bringing together young people from different backgrounds gives the organisation an energy which has sustained it.

David: Also, we have always encouraged a very friendly, informal, first name relationship between our teachers, volunteers, and youngsters. I suspect that more training and development takes place in the corridors than in the classrooms, because that's where the informal chats happen. That's where some of the most valuable life lessons can be learned.

Marian: Then there's the curriculum. It's not just about teaching magic tricks. We have many different activities, including workshops, competitions, and shows. There's also mime, clowning, puppetry, ventriloquism, juggling, and theatre production.

David: It's a very holistic approach. Nowadays people can learn magic online, but we offer something that is much more varied and interesting.

How Does It All Work?

David: The courses are offered as an extramural, after-school, activity. We enrol about 120 to 150 younger students each year and their lessons take place on a Saturday morning. The seniors will spend their Saturday afternoons here too. The seniors will also spend many afternoons here. We have around 30 volunteer teachers, including a number of experts assisting, some even via zoom. Most are graduates of our organisation who want to give something back to the community.

Marian: Giving back is very important. We organise big public shows in which the youngsters perform great illusions and magic. They love being on stage and usually want to continue appearing in future shows. But once they graduate, they are encouraged to help backstage and to train the next group of youngsters, but they can't perform in the shows. We always say to them that they have had their turn and that they have something valuable to give back.

Can You Talk About Your Work with Those from Marginalised Groups?

David: A good 60% of the students fall into that category. They come from poor areas and are being sponsored. As I mentioned earlier, the organisation is all about diversity and so we work hard to ensure that the student cohort represents all of South Africa. The legacy of apartheid means that the marginalised students often live a considerable distance from the College. They must travel for a long time to get here and those journeys have become very expensive. Plus, there are safety issues. Two years ago, one of our students was murdered, and every couple of weeks we have an incident.

Marian: Also, all the youngsters are given the same equipment, and in our competitions, they are required to perform with that apparatus. That encourages them to demonstrate their creativity and performance skills, and no one has an advantage because they can afford fancy apparatus.

David: The more privileged youngsters often receive a lot of support at home whereas this is not always the case for those from the marginalised community. That support is important and so we interview all families to check that there will be some sort of support to help sustain them. Getting that buy in from some communities can be quite a challenge because in some areas of South African people are suspicious about witchcraft and magic. But we've come a long way since the 1980s to educate our local population about the art of conjuring. The growing number of people coming to see our public shows proves that.

Can You Talk About the College's Rural Programmes?

David: Yes. These involve travelling out to youngsters who can't get to us because they live too far away. These courses last six weeks and involve our instructors going to areas that are a one-to-two-hour drive away from the College. Each week a group of youngsters have a two-hour session and these focus on learning juggling and card skills. Often the word magic isn't used there at all. Travel is expensive and so we're looking to get a sponsored vehicle next year. Our rural programmes currently reach about 320 young people and we plan to double that by 2025.

Marian: We teach them the eight 'star' qualities as well as the juggling and card skills. Over the last 10 years, we have worked hard to increase the number of girls on our courses. In some places, we have scholarships that target girls. Our rural programmes have recruited equal numbers of boys and girls, and the girls are doing incredibly well. In these poorer communities, girls were expected to do chores at home, while the boys went out and had fun. But we're encouraging more equality.

What's Special About Magic?

David: I think that's the key question. Magic is what excites the youngsters, and it has a very special energy. Also, there is always something new to learn. I've been involved with the College for 40 years and I'm still learning. Magic is also a wonderful way of creating the skills that you've identified in your work, including self-confidence and communication skills. Perhaps most important of all in the twenty-first century, magic enhances the imagination. Many of our graduates come back and tell us that they're not doing magic anymore, but that the imagination-based skills that they learned here are vital to their careers.

Then there is connectedness and conversations. In the rural communities, a child might learn a card trick, but when they go home, they've faced with alcohol abuse and other issues. But the card tricks make the father interested. Suddenly the youngster has got a power that they have never had before, and they get their attention from their father in a positive way.

Marian: Can I just add that for many years we've been waiting for magic to be recognised in the arts world. Governments often have a department of arts and culture, but they don't tend to include magic. Funders often include dance, drama, and music, but not magic. We are so excited to think that magic may finally get the recognition that it deserves.

SUMMARY

This chapter has examined how magic is used to build key life skills, including creativity (solving and inventing illusions), empathy (crafting presentations that others will enjoy), self-control (practising and rehearsing), organisation and memory (recalling the correct sequence of events), self-confidence and social skills (successfully performing an illusion), preparedness (thinking of what might go wrong during a performance), and resilience (handling disappointment when an illusion fails). This work has involved a wide range of cohorts, and research into the efficacy of this approach has generally yielded positive results.

4

PEDAGOGICAL PRESTIDIGITATION

This chapter examines the various ways in which Applied Magic is used within an educational context, including to promote learning and curiosity, to communicate science and mathematics, to enhance design and maker skills, to teach foreign languages, and to encourage scepticism about paranormal phenomena.

LEARNING AND CURIOSITY

Several articles (e.g. McCormack, 1985; Vidler & Levine, 1981) and books (Goodman & Furman, 1981; McCormack, 1990) have explored how educators can use magic to elevate flagging energy levels, to create interest, and as a reward for good behaviour. Goodman and Furman (1981) also describe how illusions can be used to promote engagement by involving shy and quiet students, to highlight the importance of listening to instructions by having students follow along with an illusion, and to help to create a positive teaching environment. Each of these ideas is illustrated with several illusions. For example, the authors describe how teachers might perform The Magic Pencil (see Chapter Two) with a ruler and then use the illusion as a catalyst to discuss the best ways of making rules stick.

Much of this work also explores how magic can be used in specific lessons, including geography, physical education, science, mathematics, social studies, art, and music. For instance, Goodman and Furman (1981) describe how geography teachers could draw a map of the world on an inflated balloon and ask their students to identify a particular country. They then stick a pin into the chosen country, and if the student is correct, the balloon doesn't burst. This illusion is achieved by secretly placing some transparent tape over the correct country. Similarly, McCormack (1990) describes how art students could make an origami rabbit magically animate its ears, and how music students could have someone secretly select a song, appear to read the person's mind, and then play the chosen song. Additional work focussing on employing magic to communicate science and mathematics will be discussed in the following section.

Outside the classroom, magicians and educational practitioners use magic to deliver information about various topics, including healthy living, dental hygiene, road safety, religion, and environmentalism. For example, during a children's show about personal hygiene, a performer might show pictures of germs, have the children pretend to wash their hands, and then show that the germs on the pictures have magically vanished. Engs (1998) used magic to deliver AIDS education to teenagers, including illusions in which the magician produces a condom from a previously empty HIV prevention pamphlet, and a version of The Twenty-One Card Trick (see Chapter One) that employs the magic phrase 'Use Condoms'. Similarly, magician Megan Swann performs a show designed to promote environmental issues. Megan received a Good Magic Award for this work in 2020 and is currently the President of The Magic Circle.

Cause for Wonder was created by magician Lisa Mena and uses magic to influence people's attitudes and behaviours about a range of social and health issues. This work involves magicians performing illusions that are designed to deliver key information and spectators repeating magical phrases that highlight these messages. For instance, to promote women's rights in India, Antigua, and Ethiopia, male spectators were asked to repeat the magic phrase 'Helping Women Brings Good Things'. These shows encourage prolonged engagement because spectators are likely to discuss them with their friends and family after the show.

In 2007, I started the Quirkology YouTube channel to encourage curiosity and critical thinking. Many of the illusion-based videos on the channel contain two sections, with the first section showing a seemingly impossible illusion and the second section revealing the secret to the illusion. These videos use new and elaborate methods that usually wouldn't work in live performances. For example, in the first part of one video, I produce a large ball from an empty cloth. In the second section, viewers discover that this illusion is the result of someone standing several metres behind me and using a long rod to secretly pass the ball to me. The videos have attracted over 500 million views, have proved popular with magicians, and are frequently used by educators. A few years ago, the British magic manufacturer Marvin's Magic produced a Quirkology optical illusion kit for the public.

I have also teamed up with sleight of hand expert Will Houstoun to create videos that celebrate scientific and technological achievements. In these videos, a narrator describes a topic and Houstoun highlights key points by performing magic with specially printed playing cards. For example, a video about the Apollo Moon landings involves the sudden appearance of a card showing the Sputnik satellite, and an illustration of the Saturn V rocket magically transforms into a picture of the Command Module. These videos have attracted over 700,000 views on YouTube.

A few years ago, I suggested that magic might form part of a school curriculum (Derbyshire, 2008; Paton, 2008), and several initiatives have recently started to explore this possibility.

In Scotland, Kevin Quantum (The Edinburgh International Magic Festival) has created an online resource for teachers wanting to perform and teach magic in their lessons. The use of branching technology allows participants to have a personalised learning experience based on the choices they make in each module, and the course aims to enhance a range of skills and abilities, including self-confidence, maker skills, numeracy, and literacy.

In England, David Brookhouse, a magician, lecturer, and manager of Heritage Learning Lancashire, is piloting a magic-based educational scheme for schoolchildren aged 7–11 years. After taking an oath of secrecy, participants are taught several illusions and encouraged to create novel presentations. They then visit a local museum or heritage site and are asked to devise some magic that helps to convey a story associated with the collection, site, or community. At the end of the project, the children present their illusions in a stage show. The project involves magician Russ Brown, and aims to promote a range of skills, including self-confidence, creativity, art, design, numeracy, and literacy. Initial feedback has been very positive, and the scheme appears to be especially helpful to children who struggle with more mainstream forms of teaching. To discover more about this work, see my interview with David later in this chapter.

Researchers have assessed the impact of magic on curiosity and learning, and generally obtained positive results.

Lustig (1994) created a magic show that aimed to inform children aged 11–14 years about AIDS. The show consisted of bespoke illusions that dispelled misconceptions about transmission of the illness and encouraged safer sex. For example, the effectiveness of condoms was illustrated by a huge needle penetrating an inflated condom without bursting it. A questionnaire administered before and after the show suggested that spectators' knowledge about AIDS was significantly increased, and that they were more confident about refusing sex and using condoms.

Liakos (2016) assessed a Cause for Wonder initiative that aimed to help villagers living by Mozambique's Lake Niassa appreciate the importance of keeping the lake clean from chemicals and human excrement. The project was carried out in collaboration with the Manda Wilderness Community Trust and involved a magician performing a bespoke show in five villages close to the lake. During the show, spectators were asked to recite the phrase 'A Clean Lake is a Happy Life', and to watch several illusions illustrating this theme. The assessment involved around 400 people, and showed that the illusions and key phrase were well remembered in the five villages, with news about the performances spreading by word of mouth to surrounding areas. In addition, people who had seen the magic show indicated that they were more likely to engage in hygienic behaviours, although some respondents noted the difficulty in changing their habits due to a lack of alternative options.

Moss et al. (2017) carried out an online study involving four groups of adults. One group was shown a video of gory magic in which a person was apparently sawn in half; a second group saw the same video but was told the secret of the illusion; a third group watched a video of a circus act and the final group acted as a control and didn't see any video at all. Participants then saw a video tutorial about neuroscience, rated their engagement with the tutorial and answered questions about its content. Those who hadn't seen either the unexplained magic or circus videos were more absorbed in the tutorial. The authors speculate that watching the magic, but not finding out the solution, could cause people to fixate on the trick and that this may decrease their focus on subsequent activities.

Elder et al. (n.d.) examined the impact of incorporating magic and optical illusions into college courses on both entrepreneurship and information systems. A lecturer performed illusions that illustrated course-related content and acted as ice-breakers. Compared to the same courses being taught without illusions, the students obtained significantly higher scores in a final test and reported higher satisfaction rates. In addition, the courses incorporating the illusions enjoyed higher attendance levels. In line with the findings of Moss et al., the authors note that some of the magic caused students to focus on trying to figure out the secret of the illusions and thus disrupted learning. They suggest minimising this issue by performing the illusions prior to a break or at the end of class.

I carried out an online study evaluating magic videos that were created with Will Houstoun (Wiseman et al., 2020). Around 200 members of the public watched science videos that either did, or did not, contain magic, and then rated how they felt about the video and completed a memory test about key information. The videos containing the magic were rated as significantly more interesting, informative, and absorbing, but did not boost recall.

Finally, Ozono et al. (2021) conducted an online study in which adults watched short videos of magic, and then rated the degree to which they thought that they knew how the illusion was achieved, and whether the videos elicited a sense of surprise, interest, and curiosity. Although there was considerable variation between participants, being fooled by an illusion was, in general, positively related to curiosity, surprise, and interest. The authors have made the clips and ratings available online.

SCIENCE, MATHEMATICS, AND COMPUTING

Some magic depends on scientific or mathematical principles. For example, Chapter One describes how static electricity can be secretly employed to make a straw revolve (The Amazing Straw), a card trick that uses mathematics to ensure that a selected card ends up in a certain position within the deck (The Twenty-One Card Trick) and a seemingly impossible feat involving topology (Through a Postcard). These types of illusions are frequently used to promote science and mathematics, and many books have examined this topic in depth (e.g. Benjamin, 2016; Diaconis & Graham, 2012; Gardner, 1961; Gibson, 1975; Mould, 2019; Mulcahy, 2013; Spangler, 2021). More recently, the same approach has been used to communicate computing and coding, including work carried out as part of the Computer Science for Fun initiative at Queen Mary University of London. For a review of this area, see Wiseman and Watt (2020).

Several researchers have examined the efficacy of this work.

Papalaskari et al. (2006) describe a project in which University staff initially worked with teenagers from diverse socio-economic backgrounds to create scientific demonstrations that could be presented in a magical context. The teenagers then performed these demonstrations to younger children aged 6–12 attending a one-day magic school. For instance, the children were assigned to different groups by shining a light through a lens and seeing which of three pictures it focussed on. The children were drawn from underprivileged backgrounds, and the project presented them with a diverse set of role models and used magic to motivate learning. It also provided the teenagers with an enjoyable enrichment activity that encouraged community engagement. An evaluation showed that the project made most of the teenagers more interested in science, but that some of the children didn't appreciate the scientific principles behind the magic. Papalaskari et al. (2007) addressed this issue in a follow-up project by having the teenagers create a booklet that explained the science behind the illusions.

Lin et al. (2014, 2017) assessed the impact of magic demonstrations in physics lessons. In one study, some students, aged 13–14 years, were taught about friction using well-known demonstrations whilst others were shown science-based magic. For example, in one lesson, the teacher threaded a plastic ball onto a piece of string and then magically made it stop and start as it slid down. This was achieved by a secret mechanism inside the ball that used friction to stop the ball's movement when the string was secretly pulled taught. The magic increased students' confidence in learning science, as well as boosting understanding and knowledge retention.

Taufiq et al. (2017) had students, aged 13–14 years, complete a physics test and then split them into two groups. One group was asked to predict the outcome of a magic demonstration. For example, the teacher burst an inflated balloon by pushing it down on an upturned nail and then asked what would happen if the balloon was pushed onto a bed of nails. After the students predicted that the nails would burst the balloon, the teacher showed that the inflated balloon remained intact. The other group saw demonstrations that didn't involve any seemingly magical events. Both groups then completed the physics test again, and those who had seen the magic demonstrations obtained significantly higher scores.

Some work has evaluated the use of magic to teach mathematics and computer science. Ferreira and Mendes (2014) included mathematical card tricks in undergraduate lectures and discovered that the students found the sessions especially engaging, motivating, and educational. Similarly, Curzon and McOwan (2008) and Curzon et al. (2009) showed that magic increased students' understanding of key concepts in computer science. Finally, Hilas and Politis (2014) used magic to teach ideas relating to computer networks, with students rating the course as highly engaging and interesting.

DESIGN AND MAKER SKILLS

Some work has examined whether magic can help designers to be more creative. Haritaipan et al. (2018a) split design students into two groups and told one group about different types of magical effects (e.g. appearances, vanishes, and levitations). All the students were then asked to create novel designs for a mug, and the designs produced by those who learned about the magical effects were judged as more creative than those in the other group. In a follow-up study, the same team found that telling the students about methods as well as effects resulted in even more creative designs (Haritaipan et al., 2018b). Similarly, Li (2020) had design students complete a creativity test in which they had to come up with unusual uses for everyday objects (the Alternative Uses Test), watch some magic, discover the methods, and then complete the test again. The students' creativity scores were significantly higher after they had been taught about magic.

Although many illusions are performed with everyday objects, some require bespoke equipment. Making this apparatus promotes a range of maker skills as it involves constructing prototypes and props from various materials, including cardboard, wood, metal, plastic, paper, and mirrors. In North America, the children's performer Mario 'the Maker' Magician uses cardboard and electronics to build props and robotic assistants for his shows and encourages audiences to engage in maker activities (Marchese, 2021a, 2021b). For more information about Mario's work, see my interview with him later in this chapter.

TEACHING FOREIGN LANGUAGES

In (2009) describes several ways in which magic can help in teaching foreign languages, including having students perform illusions to increase their vocabulary, fluency, and communication skills. In advises splitting a class into two groups, teaching a different illusion to each group, and then pairing-up students from the two groups to ensure that they can perform to someone who isn't aware of the method. In also describes how showing students an illusion, and having them write instructions for others to follow, can promote students' literacy and comprehension skills.

Adipramono and Nindhita (2016) evaluated whether this approach could help in teaching English to students in Indonesia. Students were shown several illusions and asked to explain how they thought that each one was achieved. This was seen as an enjoyable activity and helped the students to learn vocabulary. In a similar study, Ikhsanudin et al. (2019) had students watch an illusion and then listen to an audio recording describing the secret. The students were motivated to discover the secret and were therefore especially attentive to the recording.

Spencer and Balmer (2020) examined whether Kevin Spencer's Hocus Focus™ programme (see Chapter Three) could help students to learn English. The study involved junior high school students whose native languages were Spanish, Mandarin Chinese, and Portuguese. The students were asked to write presentations for several illusions and to use electronic devices to translate these scripts into English. The authors describe an overall increase in students initiating conversations in English and increased scoring on measures of self-efficacy (Self-Efficacy Scale Condensed Version), self-esteem (Rosenberg Self-Esteem Scale), and motivation (Duckworth Grit Scale).

SCEPTICISM ABOUT THE PARANORMAL PHENOMENA

Magicians have long promoted scepticism about paranormal phenomena by demonstrating and exposing the tricks used by fake psychics and mediums (for a review, see Truzzi, 1997). Several famous magicians have been involved in this work, including Harry Houdini and James Randi in America, and Derren Brown in Britain. In addition, academics with a background in magic, myself included, have used magic in talks and lectures to boost scepticism about psychic phenomena.

In an early example of this approach, Marcuse and Bitterman (1944) lectured to students about the reality of paranormal phenomena and then introduced an individual who claimed to be telepathic. This person performed several pseudo-psychic magic tricks, such as answering questions that were sealed in envelopes. Around 80% of the students indicated that they believed the demonstrations were evidence of psychic powers. The lecturer then revealed that the group had been fooled and explained the need for them to think critically about the paranormal phenomena. In a more recent example, Goodin (2010) described performing magic in lectures about paranormal phenomena and notes that around a third of students believed that these feats were the result of genuine psychic abilities. When Goodin revealed that they had been deceived, some of these students became angry whilst others continued to believe that he possessed genuine powers.

Some research works have assessed the impact of this work.

During an undergraduate course about critical thinking and paranormal phenomena, McBurney (1976) had a magician perform several seemingly psychic feats and then explain how these illusions were accomplished. McBurney didn't assess the specific impact of this demonstration, but surveys taken before and after the course indicate that the students had become more sceptical about the psychic phenomena. Similarly, Dougherty (2004) conducted two studies with undergraduate students at an American liberal arts college. Each time, one group of undergraduate students enrolled in a sceptical course on paranormal phenomena whilst others took alternative courses. Towards the start of the sceptical course, the instructor claimed to possess psychic abilities and performed various illusions to support these claims. Later in the course, the instructor revealed the secrets behind these illusions. Surveys from both studies suggested that, compared to the alternative courses, the sceptical course significantly decreased students' belief in paranormal phenomena.

In a related work, I recently teamed up with comic book writer Rik Worth and artist Jordan Culver to produce five comics that explore psychology, magic, and paranormal phenomena. Entitled *Hocus Pocus*, these comics present factual stories about seemingly psychic phenomena and often incorporate interactive illusions. We recently conducted an online study to evaluate the impact of these comics and illusions on readers' belief in the paranormal phenomena (Wiseman et al., 2021). Over 500 members of the public saw one of three versions of the comics (comic strips with an interactive illusion, comic strip without an illusion or a text-based version of the strip) and rated their level of scepticism about the psychic phenomena. The results showed that the comics were an effective way of promoting scepticism amongst those with a prior interest in comics.

PRACTITIONER INTERVIEWS

David Brookhouse

David is a magician and manager of Heritage Learning Lancashire. He is piloting a scheme that uses magic in schools to promote numeracy and literacy, to enhance other key life skills, and to boost engagement with local museums and heritage sites.

When and How Did You Get Started in Magic?

I was around 7 years old, and I was visiting a hotel in Blackpool with my grandma and mum. A magician performed a trick with some sponge balls, and I was completely mesmerised. He could see that I was really interested, and he told me about a shop selling tricks in Blackpool. My grandma and I then went there most weeks, and when I was about 15 years old, I met magic mentor Bill Thompson, and soon became one of his acolytes.

How Would You Describe Your Career and Job?

I've been in the heritage sector for about 17 years. I run a heritage, culture, and arts organisation that delivers learning to all age groups, including providing outreach for schools. It's not about telling teachers how to teach, but supporting them and providing new, dynamic, and interesting learning environments and platforms. For example, to support the history curriculum, we might send one of my team into a school as a Roman soldier. It's authentic, experiential, hands-on learning.

Where Did the Idea for Your Magic-Based Work Come from?

Magic equipped me with many essential skills, including problem-solving skills, analytical skills, social skills, and storytelling skills. Perhaps most important of all, it gave me a huge amount of self-confidence. I have always wanted others to enjoy these benefits and so I have been thinking about bringing magic into school for years. When children missed fundamental aspects of their education due to the COVID pandemic, I thought that now was the time to see if magic can help. Over the years, we have successfully run several projects as part of the Museums and Schools Programme, funded by the Department for Education and managed by the Arts Council. I teamed up with a local magician and friend, Russ Brown, and pitched a magic-based project to them. They liked the idea and agreed to support it.

How Does the Project Work?

We want to support children's numeracy and literacy levels, to help them to develop several soft skills, and to engage with their local heritage and community. We're working with 6 classes of around 30 children. Each class is from a different school. The first stage involves training the six teachers who are in charge of these classes to be comfortable and confident with magic.

So, You Are Teaching the Teachers?

Yes, teacher development is very important. We don't want teachers to feel like it this is being done to them but rather with them. We hold workshops where we teach the teachers how to perform several tricks. We're not telling them how to use the tricks, that's for them to decide. Instead, we are upskilling them so that they can use magic as an educational tool.

The six teachers have been fantastic, and they have had some very creative ideas. For example, there is one trick where a volunteer randomly pairs up playing cards from a deck and discovers that they have matched the two threes, two fours, two jacks, and so on. It can be used in history lessons as a fun way to match dates and events, or in geography to match capitals and countries.

And Then the Children Learn Magic from Both the Teachers and You?

Yes. The teachers show the children how to perform magic, and each school now has a magic club where everyone learns some tricks. Russ and I also hold workshops in each school. We perform a trick and show the children how it works. They have to write down the information in their books, including the effect, the apparatus, the mechanics, etc., that promotes literacy and problem solving. Then, we explain that they must create their own storyline and write that in their book too. This promotes creativity and imagination, and the written work that we're getting from them is phenomenal.

In addition, we have placed seven magic books in each school library, and this encourages the children to engage with books and enhances their reading skills. Some of the children have also asked older family members who happen to know some magic to teach them a trick and have brought that into school. It's been wonderful to see. One teacher told us about a child who craved attention, and performing magic allowed him to get that in a positive and appropriate way. Another said that they had a girl who sat at the back of the class and didn't like learning. But magic interests her and now she writes everything down, asks questions, and even wants to perform.

And You're Also Involving Local Museums and Heritage Sites?

Yes. Russ and I accompany the class to a local site, and the staff there take us on a tour and allow everyone to explore. The children are asked to think about how they can use magic to tell a story associated with the site. We have used music, dance, and poetry to do this in the past, but not magic. It gives everyone a very different perspective.

Even the museum and heritage staff look at their collections in a new way, so it's been good for their professional development too.

Each class then returns to school with lots of ideas and discusses them. They then choose one idea and create an illusion that helps to tell that story. At the end of the project, all six schools come together to stage a show containing these six pieces. All 300 children will be in the audience, so it's a big show. We obviously don't want to pressurise any of the children to perform, so there are opportunities for them to make apparatus, to help backstage, to control the lighting and sound, and so on.

Where Does It Go in the Future?

I would love to roll this out to other schools across the country. Maybe we will create a professional development course or a book. Teachers would love that. It all depends on funding. For me, it's about helping children and teachers. I know what magic did for me, and it would be great if this work can help others have the same enjoyment and benefits.

Also, in the same way that Bill Thompson inspired me all those years ago, I hope that this will inspire some new magicians in the future. Like any art form, magic needs young people and new ideas. If we get one or two children who continue their journey into magic, then that's a huge win for me.

Mario 'the maker' Magician

Mario creates and performs educational, inspiring, kids' shows that combine handmade apparatus and robotics. Based in New York, Mario, his wife and two children tour the country appearing at a variety of venues, including schools and maker fairs. The famous magician David Blaine has referred to him as 'the best kids' magician in the world'.

How Did You Get Started?

I hitchhiked across America when I was 17 years old. At one point, I met some kids from California, and they were paying for their trip by playing guitar on the street. It planted a seed, and I started performing on the street, mainly playing music. I eventually ended up in Michigan and went to a magic store to get some tricks for a friend. It was amazing. The store was stuffed from floor to ceiling with magic props. I learnt a few tricks and got hooked. I joined a local magic club and, in my 20s, landed my first magic job performing in a restaurant. I'm first-generation American. My father worked hard as a stonemason and didn't really enjoy what he did. That showed me the importance of having a job that you find fun. Long story short, I ended up living just outside of New York City, and there were lots of opportunities to perform magic at birthday parties. I started performing for kids, and in 2006, my wife and I took a risk and quit our day jobs. After a year or so, we were making enough to pay our rent and it's all grown from there.

What Are the Main Messages in Your Show?

My show is based around three ideas: do what you love; use what you have; and have fun.

At one point, I explain how a teacher changed my life by telling me how the famous artist Andy Warhol painted tomato cans for a living. Then I explain that he was once asked why he painted tomato cans, and he said that he just loved tomato soup! That story allows me to talk about why it's important to do what you love.

Later, I talk about how an artist named Alexander Calder borrowed broken toys from his neighbours, mixed them together and made an amazing toy that had never existed before. I ask the kids if they would like to know what he built, and when they all shout 'Yes', I talk about how he constructed an entire circus out of broken toys. It's called Calder Circus. It was the start of performance art and changed the world. That's all about using what you have.

And then there's the importance of having fun. I take out just one clown nose, and it starts multiplying. Soon they are appearing everywhere – in my glasses, on my nose, in my ears, in my hat, and so on. At the end of the show, we throw hundreds of clown noses into the audience, and everyone gets to take one home. That's a reminder to always have fun.

I Know That You Perform with Homemade Props – Can You Tell Me More About That?

That's all part of using what you have. Cardboard has become an organic theme for me. It also helps with accessibility and connecting. The kids see the cardboard props and they can relate to them. It's not like I have spent a bunch of money and bought apparatus that they have never seen before. They have made things from cardboard and so they think that they can make the same objects when they go home. There are always a few kids in the audience who get in a lot of trouble because they struggle to sit still or to contain their emotions. The cardboard props really help me to connect with them. Connection is so important to me. It's more important than the magic.

Are You Also Trying to Encourage the Kids' Maker Skills?

Yes. One of the greatest comments came from a mum who told me that her kid came home from a show and said: 'Mom. I'm going to go through the recycling and trash bin, and I'm going to make a magic show like Mario'. I thought that was great. That's where great art comes from. It doesn't matter how successful and rich you are, great art still comes from the bottom. Hip hop came from the South Bronx. The poorest of poor neighbourhoods, but it transformed the music industry!

How Did You Move into Robotics?

I have always loved making marionettes and puppets. Then, in 2005, I picked up *Make: Magazine* and there was this little blue board on the cover. You plugged it in, and you could make motors move. I spent two years learning how to code, eventually got the hang of it, and made automata for art galleries.

Next, I started to incorporate robotics into my homemade magic apparatus. During the opening of my show, two banners open and say 'Mario' and 'World's greatest'. They're robotic and involve lots of servos. Then flags come up and as I take my bow, one of the signs falls off. I fix it, take my bow and the other side goes. The next thing you know, it's chaos. Spring snakes shoot out from my case, and a cannon fires loads of ping-pong balls everywhere. Throughout the show, there's always a sense of panic because something has broken or fallen apart. Kids are used to adults telling them what to do, and so they find it refreshing to see an adult in trouble and having to deal with it.

We've also had lots of success on social media with Automabot – a cardboard robot that makes a ball of aluminium foil appear and disappear. Unfortunately, someone stole it when we were on tour, but I think it was a blessing because it's forced me to focus on my live show.

Make: Magazine has published two books of mine – one on making magic with household objects and the other focussing on robotics. I would have never dreamed that we'd be brand ambassadors for them. They inspired me and so it has come full circle.

What Are Your Thoughts About Revealing the Secrets to Some Tricks?

In the show, I have a long streamer that I wave around, and I tell the kids not to pull on it. And then I just drape the streamer through the audience, and one of the children will pull on it and rip it. I cry like a baby, grab the broken streamer, crumble it up into my hand, sprinkle some confetti and it comes out in one piece. One of my books describes how to make and perform the streamer trick. Magicians often think that's a bad idea, but I am happy to give that away because someone did that for me when I was a kid. If I didn't have someone who did that for me, maybe I wouldn't be where I am today.

But it's a gray area. Some performers are making money by revealing secrets on social media, and it can be very infuriating for creators. I totally respect that. But I think that it's important to feed breadcrumbs to your audience. For me, the streamer routine is like a breadcrumb that might encourage people to get into magic. Sometimes I get an e-mail from families who have built several items from the book and that feels amazing.

I Think We Share a Hero in Fred Rogers

I'm so glad you're asking this stuff. Just hearing his name makes me emotional. Mr Rogers encouraged people to look for a greater purpose in life and to stick with it. It's not easy to dedicate your life to lifting kids up because it's like planting trees and knowing that you're not going to sit in the shade of the tree. It's very difficult for us as humans because we want recognition and fame in our own lifetime. School shows are very humbling. It's not like being a rock star where everyone is patting you on the back. But it's beautiful to think about what you've created. How you have inspired kids to learn, to grow and be the best human they can be.

SUMMARY

Applied Magic is used in a wide range of educational settings. Teachers perform magic to promote curiosity and learning, magicians stage shows to convey key messages about road safety and healthy living, and lecturers use illusions to communicate science, mathematics, and computer science. In addition, magic can boost comprehension and communication among those learning a foreign language, enhance design and maker skills, and help to build a healthy degree of scepticism about paranormal phenomena. In general, research into the efficacy of this work has obtained positive results and supported the educational value of magic-based interventions.

CONCLUSION

Throughout the course of this book, we have explored the many ways in which Applied Magic promotes wellbeing. We took a brief glimpse into the secretive subculture of conjuring, learned about the illusions that are used in therapeutic and educational work, discovered how medical magic boosts patients' health, found out how to conjure up life skills, and investigated how prestidigitation enhances learning. Along the way, we surveyed key initiatives from around the world, explored research examining the efficacy of this work, and encountered in-depth interviews with experienced performers and practitioners.

We discovered how magic is used by a wide range of practitioners (including teachers, physicians, nurses, occupational therapists, counsellors, and social workers), helps lots of people (including hospital patients, children undergoing counselling, individuals with learning differences, young adults at risk from gang violence, and those marginalised within society), involves a variety of interventions (including individual and group work, and short performances to lengthy courses), and results in many important benefits (including increased confidence, better social skills, higher levels of creativity, and improved coordination). Together, this vast amount of material demonstrates the power, practicality, and flexibility of Applied Magic to promote physical and psychological health.

TOWARDS THE FUTURE

This section outlines seven ways in which Applied Magic may develop in the future.

One: Although past initiatives have involved a diverse range of cohorts, surprisingly little work has specifically targeted older people (although see Lee et al., 2022a, b). This is unfortunate as many countries have an ageing population, with older people often experiencing a range of challenges, including poor mental health, mobility problems, loneliness, and ageism. Future work could examine the potential beneficial effects of teaching older people magic, including increased intergenerational connectivity, raised self-esteem, and slower cognitive decline.

Two: Most interventions have been carried out face to face, with only a small amount of work exploring whether the same effects can be obtained using digital delivery (e.g. live online platforms, mobile phones, and pre-recorded videos). This bias is understandable, given that magic is best seen live and teaching people to perform illusions often involves showing them how to carry out certain movements. However, digital delivery clearly offers the potential for increased scalability and greater geographical reach. Those interested in the approach may benefit from studying how magicians moved their shows online during the COVID-19 pandemic, including how they used interactive illusions, created apparatus that could be sent to participants prior to the show, and employed multiple cameras to provide viewers with a more immersive experience (Gareth, 2020; Houstoun & Thompson, 2020).

Three: Several psychologists, myself included, have argued for better quality research (e.g. Bagienski & Kuhn, 2019, 2020; Wiseman & Watt, 2018, 2020). There is the potential for a range of improvements, including future researchers employing larger sample sizes, using control groups, comparing the impact of magic to other activities, tracking the effect of interventions over longer periods of time, pre-registering studies, and moving away from self-report measures and towards real-world indicators of success and wellbeing (e.g. physical health, exam results, and employment history).

Four: Future work could benefit from being informed by relevant theories from academic psychology. For example, Seligman (2012) suggested that wellbeing can be understood through the lens of the PERMA model (Positive emotions, Engagement and absorption,

Relationships and connectivity, Meaningful activity, and Accomplishment) and, within an educational context, Dweck (2007) has written about the importance of a Growth Mindset (a belief that people can change through hard work and dedication). I have written about the application of the Growth Mindset to magic (Wiseman & Kaye, 2020), and Bagienski and Kuhn (2019, 2020) have explored the PERMA model. This approach will benefit from identifying and classifying the various benefits of watching and performing magic. Bagienski and Kuhn have argued that such benefits fall into four categories, and my approach is presented in Appendix 2 and involves five categories (Watching magic, Being interested in magic, Creating magic, Practicing magic, and Performing magic).

Five: Future work could further explore some of the novel uses of magic identified in the previous chapters. Possible candidates for topics could include investigating how hospital magic has a positive effect on patients' siblings, how creating plots and presentations fosters imagination and creativity, how health professionals can use magic to help carry out treatments and procedures, how magic provides people with a new and positive topic of conversation, and how writing the instructions for illusions encourages perspective taking and communication skills.

Six: When developing new interventions, it would be helpful to focus on what is unique about magic. Several academics have explored why magic is unlike other performing arts, with much of this work noting that during a magic show, spectators do not have to suspend their disbelief and instead see a seemingly impossible event happening right in front of their eyes (e.g. Lamont, 2017; Leddington, 2016). Future work could explore the therapeutic and educational benefits of this unique experience, including how magic helps to generate awe and astonishment, awaken hope, and encourage a more expansive mindset.

Seven: Future work could examine how work in magic and wellbeing can improve the art of conjuring. The Argentinian magician René Lavand lost his hand at an early age and so had to invent new methods and presentations. As a result, he is now widely considered to have been one of the most innovative and creative magicians in the world. Similarly, the limitations associated with therapeutic and educational magic could help to change and improve the art of magic. Also, some magicians perform to show off and to boost their ego, whilst Applied Magic focuses on helping others. Encouraging magicians to think about ways in which audiences could benefit from their performances may result in more meaningful illusions and presentations.

A FINAL THOUGHT

I hope that you have enjoyed our sojourn into the world of Applied Magic. This work has touched the lives of countless people across the globe and helped to make the world a better place. Regardless of whether you are already working in this area, or thinking about becoming involved, I hope that this book will inspire you to bring a much-needed sense of wonder to even more people and to celebrate what I and many other magicians consider to be the real magic of magic.

APPENDIX 1
ADDITIONAL RESOURCES

RECOMMENDED READING

Each chapter has referenced specialised manuals and books about Applied Magic. Here are some additional books that are aimed at beginners and explore the psychology and history of magic.

Books for Beginners

Pogue, D. (1998). *Magic for dummies.* IDG Books Worldwide Inc. Describes many great effects along with interesting discussions about performing magic.

Wilson, M. (1988). *Mark Wilson's complete course in magic.* Running Press.
A classic volume describing hundreds of tricks, including close-up magic, mind reading, and stage illusions.

Einhorn, N. (2009). *The illustrated compendium of magic tricks.* Lorenz Books.
Contains thousands of photographs and hundreds of tricks that are suitable for beginners.

Kronzek, A. Z. (2018). *Grandpa magic.* Workman Publishing.
One of the few books that is aimed to older people wanting to perform magic.

Ackerly, P. (2020). *Magic tricks for kids*. Rockridge Press.
An inexpensive and clear book of magic for young people.

Edmonson, M., & Parsons, G. (2017). *The greatest magician in the world*. Macmillan.
A beautifully illustrated and highly creative book that combines storytelling and magic.

Jay, J. (2014). *Big magic for little hands*. Workman Publishing.
A lovely big book for children, containing clear instructions and some great magic.

History of Magic

Copperfield, D., Wiseman, R., Britland, D., & Liwag, H. (2021). *David Copperfield's history of magic*. Simon & Schuster.
This lavishly illustrated book explores the history of conjuring through David Copperfield's secret museum of magic.

Lamont, P., & Steinmeyer, J. (2018). *The secret history of magic: The true story of a deceptive art*. Tarcher Perigee.
A thorough and academic guide to history and magic.

Psychology and Magic

Lamont, P., & Wiseman, R. (1999). *Magic in theory: An introduction to the theoretical and psychological elements of conjuring*. University of Hertfordshire Press.
How magicians perceive the psychology of conjuring.

Kuhn, G. (2019). *Experiencing the impossible: The science of magic*. MIT Press.
A comprehensive overview of research into the psychology of magic.

MAGAZINES AND WEBSITES

The following magazines and websites provide up to date information about the world of magic.

Genii, The Conjurors' Magazine: www.geniimagazine.com
This long running and glossy American monthly magazine is
essential reading for anyone interested in magic.

Magicseen: www.magicseen.com
A British magazine contain articles about the latest developments
in magic and interviews with leading performers.

Vanish: www.vanishmagic.com
A monthly magazine containing lots of tricks, reviews, essays,
and features.

Magic Week: www.magicweek.co.uk
Created by my old pal Duncan Trillo over 20 years ago, this wonderful website provides weekly news about magic in the UK.

MAGIC SHOPS

Search online to discover your nearest magic shop. In addition,
here are some well-known shops in Britain and America.

Britain

International Magic (London): www.internationalmagic.com
Merlins of Wakefield (Wakefield): www.merlinswakefield.co.uk
Tam Shepherds Trick Shop (Glasgow): www.tamshepherds.com
PropDog (Hounslow): www.propdog.co.uk
Alakazam (Ashford): www.alakazam.co.uk
Marvin's Magic (Hertfordshire): www.marvinsmagic.com

America

Tannen's Magic Shop (New York): www.tannens.com
Magic Inc. (Chicago): www.magicinc.net
Abbott's Magic Company (Colon): www.abbottmagic.com
Penguin Magic (online only): www.penguinmagic.com
Vanishing Inc. (online only): www.vanishingincmagic.com

ORGANISATIONS

Search online to discover your nearest local magic club. In addition, here are some national and international organisations that are based in Britain and America.

The Magic Circle: www.themagiccircle.co.uk
Founded in 1905, this British organisation holds regular meetings, lectures, and shows. Members receive a copy of *The Magic Circular* magazine and the club also supports a junior branch called the Young Magicians Club.

The Society of American Magicians: www.magicsam.com
Founded in 1902, S.A.M. describes itself as 'the oldest and most prestigious magical society in the world'. It produces *M-U-M* magazine (Magic Unity Might) and runs The Society of Young Magicians.

International Brotherhood of Magicians: www.magician.org
The largest magic organisation in the world, with around 15,000 members, and over 300 local groups in more than 80 countries. Its monthly magazine, *The Linking Ring*, contains tricks, news and reports of the groups' shows and events.

The Magic Castle: www.magiccastle.com
This private club is located in Hollywood and contains several theatres, bars, a dining room, and numerous bars. It acts as a meeting place for magicians and is home to The Academy of Magical Arts.

APPENDIX 2
36 WAYS IN WHICH MAGIC PROMOTES HEALTH AND WELLBEING

WATCHING MAGIC

Receiving attention: When people watch magic, they receive the performer's attention and if they help during a show, they become the centre of attention.

Mood: Most people like magic. As a result, watching a trick is a quick and effective way of promoting positive mood and energising a group.

Curiosity: When people see a magic show, they frequently think about how illusions might have been achieved, and this creates a sense of curiosity.

Interest: The surprising nature of magic generates interest and makes people more cognitively alert.

Awe and astonishment: Seeing a seemingly impossible event encourages an expansive mindset and evokes a sense of wonder.

Connectivity: Watching magic gives people a novel and positive topic of conversation and provides groups with a shared experience that encourages discussion.

Distraction: The absorbing nature of magic helps people to pass time in a fun way, distracts them away from concerns and worriers, and can lower pain and anxiety during medical treatment.

Empathy: Watching magic provides people with an opportunity to be a supportive audience and, on occasion, to provide a positive and constructive feedback.

Effective messaging: Magic can be used to deliver messages in a compelling and memorable way, including those associated with healthy living, science, road safety, and environmentalism.

Scepticism: Magic can help people be sceptical about alleged paranormal experiences, and about those who purport to possess magic powers (e.g. psychics, mediums, and cult leaders).

Treatment and diagnosis: Health professionals can use magic to introduce apparatus in a light-hearted and interesting way, and to help to carry out diagnoses and treatments.

BEING INTERESTED IN MAGIC

Connectivity: Developing an interest in magic brings people into contact with other like-minded individuals, and this helps to boost social support and to prevent loneliness. It can also help them to connect with friends and family by providing a new and positive topic of conversation.

Self-esteem: Being trusted with the secrets to magic tricks, and knowing something that others do not know, boosts self-esteem.

History and heritage: Magicians preserve and celebrate their past. Developing an interest in the field results in an increased understanding of social history, culture, and heritage.

Absorption: Learning about magic is an absorbing and enjoyable activity, and so helps to distract attention away from worries and concerns.

Literacy: Magicians have produced a vast literature about their art, and reading this material promotes literacy skills.

Lifelong learning: Magicians are constantly inventing new effects, methods, and presentations, and so there is always something novel to discover.

Creative problem solving: Learning methods promotes lateral and creative thinking and illustrates how apparently complex problems can have simple solutions. Also, some tricks encourage people to think about science, technology, and mathematics.

Making a meaningful contribution: The relatively small size of the magic community makes it possible for individuals to make a meaningful contribution to the future of the art by sharing their ideas with others and/or publishing them.

Personal strengths: The complex subculture of magic allows people to utilise their psychological strengths. This might involve helping with an organisation, collecting and collating historical material, inventing magic, or performing.

CREATING MAGIC

Growth mindset: Thinking about possible magical effects promotes a growth mindset because it encourages people to consider seemingly impossible and alternative possibilities.

Creative problem solving: Developing and refining methods entails creative thinking and practical problem solving. Some methods also encourage an understanding of science, mathematics, and technology.

Imagination: Inventing an interesting plot or presentation, and writing a script, promotes imagination and storytelling.

Maker skills: Creating and decorating apparatus and working with various materials promotes maker skills.

Empathy: Creating interesting effects, convincing methods, and entertaining presentations encourages people to see the world through the eyes of others, and also helps to enrich their lives.

PRACTICING MAGIC

Motor skills: Magic is a hands-on activity, and so helps to enhance fine and gross motor skills and to improve coordination.

Mastery: Many magic tricks can be learnt quite easily and so create a sense of mastery. Other tricks are more challenging and learning these generates a sense of accomplishment.

Self-control: Practicing magic helps to overcome impulsivity and promotes concentration, persistence, focus, discipline, and self-control.

Organisation and memory: Learning magic involves remembering the correct sequence of events and a script. This encourages good organisation skills and memory.

Preparedness: Thinking about what may go wrong during a performance, and how to avoid and cope with these issues, encourages preparedness.

PERFORMING MAGIC

Rapport and connectivity: Performing magic helps to develop social skills, including taking control, respecting boundaries, establishing eye contact, giving clear instructions, and overcoming nervousness. Magic also acts a catalyst to social interaction because people frequently ask to see a trick.

Confidence: A successful performance enhances people's confidence and self-esteem, and allows them to do something that others cannot do.

Adaptability and resilience: Performing magic involves adapting tricks to a given situation, dealing with unexpected events, and coping when something doesn't go to plan. This builds flexibility and resilience, and often illustrates how humour can be used to deal with anxiety.

Control: Hospital patients often feel powerless because they must undergo prescribed treatments and follow medical advice.

Performing magic provides them with a safe way of exerting control.

Team building and trust: Staging a show and performing some types of magic (e.g. double acts and illusions involving stooges) involves people working together and so encourages teamwork and trust.

Preventing burnout: Performing magic can be fun and interesting for health and educational practitioners, and thus lowers the likelihood of them experiencing stress and burnout.

REFERENCES

Adipramono, R., & Nindhita, J. (2016). The implementation of magic tricks in collaborative English learning. In *Proceedings from ICLICE 2016: The third international conference on language, innovation, culture and education* (pp. 87–92).

Bagienski, S. (2016). *The magic effects of active constructive responding on positive affect*. Dissertation completed in fulfilment of the MSc Psychology, University of Derby.

Bagienski, S. E., & Kuhn, G. (2019). The crossroads of magic and Wellbeing: A review of wellbeing-focused magic programs, empirical studies, and conceivable theories. *International Journal of Wellbeing*, 9(2), 41–65.

Bagienski, S. E., & Kuhn, G. (2020). Beyond the crossroads of magic, health, and well-being. *Public Health Panorama*, 6(1), 155–171.

Bagienski, S. E., & Kuhn, G. (2022). Supporting the psychological health of our students: An arts-based community magic workshop for adapting to university life. *Psychology of Consciousness: Theory, Research, and Practice*, 9(3), 285–303.

Bagienski, S. E., Kuhn, G., Goddard, L., & de Almeida e Souza Brodtkorb, S. (2022). Mastering the impossible: Piloting an easier-than-expected magic intervention that acts as a source of self-efficacy. *Psychology of Consciousness: Theory, Research, and Practice*, 9(3), 243–256.

Benjamin, A. (2016). *The magic of math: Solving for x and figuring out why*. Basic Books.

Binet, A. (1894). Psychology of prestidigitation. In *Annual report of the board of regents of the Smithsonian institution* (pp. 555–571). Government Printing Office.

Bonete, S., Osuna, Á., Molinero, C., & García-Font, I. (2021). MAGNITIVE: Effectiveness and feasibility of a cognitive training program through magic tricks for children with attention deficit and hyperactivity disorder. A second clinical trial in community settings. *Frontiers in Psycholology, 12*, 649527.

Bowman, R. P. (1986). The magic counsellor: Using magic tricks as tools to teach children guidance lessons. *Elementary School Guidance and Counselling, 21*, 128–138.

Bowman, R. P. (2004). *The magic counsellor: The 25 best purchasable magic tricks with unforgettable guidance lessons for kids.* Chapin.

Broome, S. A. (1995). Magic in the classroom. *Beyond Behavior: A Magazine Exploring Behavior in our Schools, 6*(2), 23–26.

Clerici, C. A., Pagani Bagliacca, E., Silva, M., Chopard, S., Puma, N., Bergamaschi, L., Gattuso, G., Sironi, G., Massimino, M., & Ferrari, A. (2021). Illusionist techniques as a complement to psychological support for children with cancer. *Tumori, 107*(2), 171–174.

Copperfield, D., & Kaufman, R. (2002). *David Copperfield's project magic handbook.* David Copperfield's Project Magic Fund, Inc.

Curzon, P., & McOwan, P. W. (2008). Engaging with computer science through magic shows. In *Proceedings of ITiCSE 2008, the 13th annual conference on innovation and technology in computer science education ACM SIGCSE* (pp. 179–183).

Curzon, P., McOwan, P. W., & Black, J. (2009). The magic of HCI: Enthusing kids in playful ways to help solve the Computer Science recruitment problem. In *Proceedings of HCI educators 2009 – playing with our education.*

Derbyshire, D. (2008, September 11). And after maths, we have magic tricks! *The Daily Mail*, 12.

Diaconis, P., & Graham, R. (2012). *Magical mathematics: The mathematical ideas that animate great magic tricks.* Princeton University Press.

Dougherty, M. J. (2004). Educating believers: Research demonstrates that courses in skepticism can effectively decrease belief in the paranormal. *Skeptic, 10*(4), 31–35.

Draklof. (1915a). *Tricks for the Trenches and Wards: Series 1: Tricks with hands and string.* Jarrold & Sons.

Draklof. (1915b). *Tricks for the Trenches and Wards: Series 2: Tricks with matches, coins and cards.* Jarrold & Sons.

Dweck, C. (2007). *Mindset: The new psychology of success.* Ballentine Books.

Elder, K. L., Deviney, D. E., MacKinnon, R. J., & Dyer, J. (n.d.). *Using illusions in the classroom: Principles, best practices, and measurement* [Unpublished manuscript]. http://www.aabri.com/SA12Manuscripts/SA12115.pdf

Elkin, D. J., & Pravder, H. D. (2018). Bridging magic and medicine. *Lancet, 391*(10127), 1254–1255.

Engs, R. C. (1998). Using magic for AIDS prevention: Some teaching techniques. *Journal of Health Education, 29*(1), 43–45.

Ezell, D., & Klein-Ezell, C. E. (2003). M.A.G.I.C. W.O.R.K.S (motivating activities geared-to instilling confidence-wonderful opportunities to raise kid's self-esteem). *Education and Training in Developmental Disabilities, 38*(4), 441–450.

Fancourt, D., Wee, J., & Lorencatto, F. (2020). Identifying mechanisms of change in a magic-themed hand-arm bimanual intensive therapy programme for children with unilateral spastic cerebral palsy: A qualitative study using behaviour change theory, *BMC Pediatrics, 20*(1), 363.

Ferreira, J. F., & Mendes, A. (2014). The magic of algorithm design and analysis: Teaching algorithmic skills using magic card tricks. In *Proceedings of the 2014 conference on innovation & technology in computer science education (ITiCSE '14) ACM* (pp. 75–80).

Gardner, M. (1961). *Entertaining mathematical puzzles.* Dover Publications.

Gareth, M. (2020). *The best balloon dog in the world.* Gareth Peter White.

Gareth, M. (2021). *On stage, online: A handbook on the virtual magic show for family entertainers.* Gareth Peter White.

Geens, A. (2005). *Project Magic: A magic project with children suffering from cancer* [Unpublished thesis]. http://www.projectmagicbelgium.be/pdf/eindwerk_anoek_geens_eng.pdf

Gibson, W. B. (1975). *Magic with science.* Putnam Publishing Group.

Gilroy, B. D. (1998). *Counseling kids: It's magic: Therapeutic uses of magic with children and teens.* Therapist Organizer.

Goodin, P. (2010). A magician in the classroom. *Skeptic, 15*(4), 38–39.

Goodman, J., & Furman, I. (1981). *Magic and the educated rabbit.* Instructo/McGraw-Hill Inc.

Green, D., Schertz, M., Gordon, A. M., Moore, A., Margalit, T. S., Farquharson, Y., Bashat, D. B., Weinstein, M., Lin, J.-P., & Fattal-Valevski, A. (2013). A multi-site study of functional outcomes following a themed approach to hand–arm bimanual intensive therapy for children with hemiplegia. *Developmental Medicine & Child Neurology, 55*(6), 527–533.

Green, D., Schertz, M., Gordon, A. M., Moore, A., Margalit, T. S., Farquharson, Y., Bashat, D. B., Weinstein, M., Lin, J.-P., & Fattal-Valevski, A. (2016). A multi-site study of functional outcomes following a themed approach to hand–arm bimanual intensive therapy for children with hemiplegia: Erratum. *Developmental Medicine & Child Neurology, 58*(3), 316.

Greve, M. (2020). *I do believe in magic.* The Magic Care Foundation.

Haritaipan, L., Saijo, M., & Mougenot, C. (2018a). Leveraging creativity of design students with a magic-based inspiration tool. In *DS 93: proceedings of the 20th international conference on engineering and product design education (E & PDE 2018)* (pp. 265–270).

Haritaipan, L., Saijo, M., & Mougenot, C. (2018b). Impact of technical information in magic-based inspiration tools on novice designers. *International Journal of Technology and Design Education, 29*(5), 1153–1177.

Hart, R., & Walton, M. (2010). Magic as a therapeutic intervention to promote coping in hospitalized pediatric patients. *Continuing Nursing Education, 36*(1), 11–16.

Hilas, C. S., & Politis, A. (2014). Motivating students' participation in a computer networks course by means of magic, drama and games. *SpringerPlus, 3*, 362.

Hines, A., Bundy, A. C., Black, D., Haertsch, M., & Wallen, M. (2019). Upper limb function of children with unilateral cerebral palsy after a magic-themed HABIT: A pre-post-study with 3- and 6-month follow-up. *Physical and Occupational Therapy in Pediatrics, 39*(4), 404–419.

Hines, A., Bundy, A. C., Haertsch, M., & Wallen, M. (2018). A magic-themed upper limb intervention for children with unilateral cerebral palsy: The perspectives of parents. *Developmental Neurorehabilitation, 22*(2), 104–110.

Houstoun, W., & Thompson, S. (2020). *Video chat magic.* Vanishing Inc.

Howard, T. W. (1977). *How to use magic in psychotherapy with children.* The Emerald Press.

Ikhsanudin, I., Sudarsono, S., & Salam, U. (2019). Using magic trick problem-based activities to improve students' engagement in a listening class. *Journal of English Language Teaching Innovation and Materials, 1,* 7–15.

In, V. (2009). Using origami and magic tricks to teach English. *The Internet TESL Journal, 15*(2). http://iteslj.org/Techniques/In-Origami.html

Jastrow, J. (1896). Psychological notes upon sleight-of-hand experts. *Science, 3,* 685–689.

Johnston, R. (2016). Discover magic...with magic! *Magic Magazine, 25*(7), 56–61.

Kelley, D. (1940). Conjuring as an asset to occupational therapy. *Occupational Therapy and Rehabilitation, 19*(1), 71–108.

Kimlat, A. (2022). *Hocus pocus practice focus: The making of a magician.* Floating Match Press.

Kuhn, G. (2019). *Experiencing the Impossible: The Science of Magic.* The MIT Press.

Kwong, E., & Cullen, N. (2007). Magic and acquired brain injury. *Canadian Association of Physical Medicine and Rehabilitation 2007 Annual Scientific Meeting.*

Labrocca, G., & Piacentini, E. O. (2015). Efficacy of magic tricks on venipuncture pain: A quasi-experimental study. *Children's Nurses: Italian Journal of Pediatric Nursing Science, 7*(1), 4–5.

Lam, M. T., Lam, H. R., & Chawla, L. (2017). Application of magic in healthcare: A scoping review. *Complementary Therapies in Clinical Practice, 26,* 5–11.

Lamont, P. (2017). A particular kind of wonder: The experience of magic past and present. *Review of General Psychology, 21,* 1–8.

Lamont, P., & Wiseman, R. (1999). *Magic in Theory: An introduction to the theoretical and psychological elements of conjuring.* University of Hertfordshire Press.

Lamont, P., & Wiseman, R. (2003). Seeing and Believing. *Magic: The Magazine for Magicians, 13*(3), 86–87.

Leddington, J. (2016). The Experience of Magic. *Journal of Aesthetics and Art Criticism, 74*(3), 253–264.

Lee, K. T., Wang, W. L., Lin, W. C., Yang, Y. C., & Tsai, C. L. (2022a). The Effects of a Magic Intervention Program on Cognitive Function and Neurocognitive Performance in Elderly Individuals With Mild Cognitive Impairment. *Frontiers in aging neuroscience, 14,* 854984.

Lee, K. T., Wang, W. L., & Yang, C. L. (2022b). Impact of a magic recreation program on older adults with minor depressive symptoms in a long-term care facility: A pilot randomized controlled trial. *Geriatric nursing, 48,* 169–176.

Levin, D. (2007). Magic arts counselling: The tricks of illusion as intervention. *Georgia School Counselors Association Journal, 23,* 14–23.

Li, T. (2020). Use of magic performance as a schema disruption method to facilitate flexible thinking. *Thinking Skills and Creativity, 38*(1), 100735.

Liakos, K. (2016). 'A clean lake is a happy life': Assessing the impact of using a magic show with a jingle and storytelling to teach water conservation issues to rural communities of Lake Niassa, Mozambique. The Liakos Group.

Lin, J., Cheng, M., Chang, Y., Li, H., Chang, J., & Lin, D. (2014). Learning activities that combine science magic activities with the 5E instructional model to influence secondary-school students' attitudes to science. *Eurasia Journal of Mathematics, Science and Technology Education, 10,* 415–426.

Lin, J., Cheng, M., Lin, S., Chang, J., Chang, Y., Li, H., & Lin, D. (2017). The effects of combining inquiry-based teaching with science magic on the learning outcomes of a friction unit. *Journal of Baltic Science Education, 16*, 218–227.

Lopez, B. (1957). Magical therapy: How the art can serve the handicapped and disturbed. *M-U-M Magazine, 46*, 445–447.

Lustig, S. L. (1994). The AIDS prevention magic show: Avoiding the tragic with magic. *Public Health Reports, 109*, 162–167.

Lyons, M., & Menolotto, A. M. (1990). Use of magic in psychiatric occupational therapy: Rationale, results and recommendations. *Australian Occupational Therapy Journal, 37*, 79–83.

Marchese, M. (2021a). *The maker magician's handbook: A beginner's guide to magic + making*. Maker Media.

Marchese, M. (2021b). *Robot magic: Beginner robotics for the maker and magician*. Maker Media.

Marcuse, F. L., & Bitterman, M. E. (1944). A classroom demonstration of 'psychical phenomena.' *The Journal of Abnormal and Social Psychology, 39*(2), 238–243.

McBurney, D. H. (1976). ESP in the psychology curriculum. *Teaching of Psychology, 3*, 66–69.

McCormack, A. J. (1985). Teaching with magic: Easy ways to hook your class on science. *Learning, 14*, 62–67.

McCormack, A. J. (1990). *Magic and showmanship for teachers*. An Ideas Factory Production.

Moss, S. A., Irons, M., & Boland, M. (2017). The magic of magic: The effect of magic tricks on subsequent engagement with lecture material. *British Journal of Educational Psychology, 87*, 32–42.

Mould, S. (2019). *Science is magic: Amaze your friends with spectacular science experiments*. DK Children.

Mulcahy, C. (2013). *Mathematical card magic: Fifty-two new effects*. AK Peters/CRC.

O'Rourke, S., Spencer, K., & Kelly, F. (2018). Development and psychometric investigation of an arts integrated assessment instrument for educators. *Journal for Learning Through the Arts, 14*(1).

Ozono, H., Komiya, A., Kuratomi, K., & Hatano, A. (2021). Magic Curiosity Arousing Tricks (MagicCATs): A novel stimulus collection to induce epistemic emotions. *Behavoural Research Methods, 53*, 188–215.

Papalaskari, M. A., Hess, K., Kossman, D., Metzger, S., Phares, A., Styer, R., Titone, C., Way, T., Weinstein, R., & Wunderlich, F. (2006). PIVOTS: Service learning at the science, theatre & magic boundary. In *Proceedings of the 36th annual frontiers in education conference. San Diego, CA: IEEE* (pp. 18–23).

Papalaskari, M. A., Hess, K., Lagalante, A., Nadi, N., Styer, R., Way, T., & Weinstein, R. (2007). Work in progress – Engineering the magic school creativity and innovation in context. In *Proceedings of the 37th annual frontiers in education conference-global engineering: knowledge without borders, opportunities without passports. IEEE* (pp. S2B1–S2B2).

Paton, G. (2008, September 11). Harry Potter-style magic lessons 'should be taught in schools'. *The Daily Telegraph*, 13.

Peretz, B., & Gluck, G. (2005). Magic trick: A behavioural strategy for the management of strong-willed children. *International Journal of Paediatric Dentistry, 15*(6), 429–436.

Pravder, H. D., Elkin, D. J., Post, S. G., & Chitkara, M. B. (2022). An innovative program using magic to provide early clinical experiences for preclinical medical students: Goals, experiences, and results of the MagicAid Program. *Medical Science Educator, 32*(1), 111–120.

Pravder, H. D., Leng-Smith, A., Brash, A. I., & Elkin, D. J. (2019). A magic therapy program to alleviate anxiety in pediatric inpatients. *Hospital Pediatrics, 9*, 942–948.

Schertz, M., Shiran, S. I., Myers, V., Weinstein, M., Fattal-Valevski, A., Artzi, M., Ben Bashat, D., Gordon, A. M., & Green, D. (2016). Imaging predictors of improvement from a motor learning-based intervention for children with unilateral cerebral palsy. *Neurorehabilitation and Neural Repair, 30*(7), 647–660.

Seligman, M. E. (2012). *Flourish: A visionary new understanding of happiness and well-being*. Atria Paperback.

Spangler, S. (2021). *Super-cool science experiments for kids: 50 mind-blowing stem projects you can do at home*. Media Lab Books.

Spencer, K. (2012). Hocus focus: evaluating the academic and functional benefits of integrating magic tricks in the classroom. *Journal of the International Association of Special Education, 13*, 87–99.

Spencer, K. W., & Balmer, S. (2020). A pilot study: Magic Tricks in the ELL classroom increasing verbal communication initiative and self-efficacy. *English Language Teaching and Linguistics Studies, 2*(1), 11–32.

Spencer, K., Yuen, H. K., Darwin, M., Jenkins, G., & Kirklin, K. (2019). Development and validation of the hocus focus magic performance evaluation scale for health professions personnel in the United States. *Journal of Educational Evaluation for Health Professions, 16*, 8.

Spencer, K., Yuen, H., Jenkins, G., Kirklin, K., & Edwards, L. (2022). A magic trick training program to improve social skills and self-esteem in adolescents with autism spectrum disorder. *American Journal of Occupational Therapy, 77*(1), 7701205120.

Spencer, K., Yuen, H., Jenkins, G., Kirklin, K., Griffin, A., Vogtle, L., & Davis, D. (2020). Evaluation of a magic camp for children with hemiparesis: A pilot study. *Occupational Therapy in Health Care, 34*(2), 155–170.

Spruill, D. A., & Poidevant, J. M. (1993). Magic and the school counselor. *Elementary School Guidance & Counseling, 27*, 229–231.

Stehouwer, R. S. (1983). Using magic to establish rapport and improve motivation in psychotherapy with children. *Psychotherapy in Private Practice, 1*(2), 85–94.

Sui, P., & Sui, M. (2007). Use of magic: Creative means for psychosocial rehabilitation. In *International health and mental health conference,* Hong Kong.

Taufiq, M., Suhandi, A., & Liliawati, W. (2017). Effect of science magic applied in interactive lecture demonstrations on conceptual understanding. *AIP Conference Proceedings 1868*, 070007-1-070007-5.

Tokar, S., & Carroll, H. J. (2004). *Side-Fx: Clinically relevant magic tricks and effects for the health-care provider.* Corporate-Fx.

Truzzi, M. (1997). Reflections on the sociology and social psychology of conjurors and their relations with psychical research. In S. Krippner (Ed.), *Advances in parapsychological research* (Vol. 8, pp. 221–271). McFarland & Company.

Vidler, D. C., & Levine, J. (1981). Curiosity, magic and the teacher. *Education, 101*, 273–275.

Weinstein, M., Myers, V., Green, D., Schertz, M., Shiran, S. I., Geva, R., Artzi, M., Gordon, A. M., Fattal-Valevski, A., & Ben Bashat, D. (2015). Brain plasticity following intensive bimanual therapy in children with hemiparesis: Preliminary evidence. *Neural Plasticity*, *2015*, 798481.

Wiseman, R., & Kaye, D. (2020). Positive magic for children. *European Journal of Applied Positive Psychology*, *4*(17), 1–4.

Wiseman, R., & Lamont, P. (2003). Déjà Vu color changing deck. *Magic: The Magazine for Magicians*, *13*(3), 87–88.

Wiseman, R., & Morris, R. L. (1995). Recalling pseudo-psychic demonstrations. *British Journal of Psychology*, *86*, 113–125.

Wiseman, R., & Watt, C. (2018). Achieving the impossible: A review of magic-based interventions and their effects on wellbeing, *PeerJ*, *6*, e6081.

Wiseman, R., & Watt, C. (2020). Conjuring cognition: A review of educational magic-based interventions. *PeerJ*, *8*, e8747.

Wiseman, R., & Watt, C. (2022). Experiencing the impossible and creativity: A targeted literature review. *PeerJ*, *10*, e13755.

Wiseman, R., Collver, J., Worth, R., & Watt, C. (2021). Hocus Pocus: Using comics to promote skepticism about the paranormal. *JCOM*, *20*(02), A04.

Wiseman, R., Greening, E., & Smith, M. (2003). Belief in the paranormal and suggestion in the seance room. *British Journal of Psychology*, *94*(3), 285–297.

Wiseman, R., Houstoun, W., & Watt, C. (2020). Pedagogic prestidigitation: Using magic tricks to enhance educational videos. *PeerJ*, *8*, e9610.

Wiseman, R., Way, D., & Foreman, G. (2022). Magic, gangs and prison. *The Psychologist*, *37*(3), 30–34.

Wiseman, R., Wiles, A., & Watt, C. (2021). Conjuring up creativity: The effect of performing magic tricks on divergent thinking. *PeerJ*, *9*, e11289.

Yuen, H. K., Spencer, K., Kirklin, K., Edwards, L., & Jenkins, G. R. (2021). Contribution of a virtual magic camp to enhancing self-esteem in children with ADHD: A pilot study. *Health Psychology Research*, *9*(1), 26986.

Yuen, H., & Spencer, K. (2019). Content validation of a checklist to evaluate therapists' competency in delivering magic tricks. *International Journal of Applied Arts Studies*, *3*(4), 77–82.